Pediatric
Nutrition Handbook

Pediatric
Nutrition Handbook

Jil Feldhausen, MS, RD

Cynthia Thomson, MS, RD, CNSD

Burris Duncan, MD

Douglas Taren, PhD

Chapman & Hall Nutrition Handbooks 3

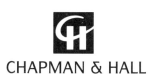

CHAPMAN & HALL

New York • Albany • Bonn • Boston • Cincinnati • Detroit • London • Madrid • Melbourne
Mexico City • Pacific Grove • Paris • San Francisco • Singapore • Tokyo • Toronto • Washington

Cover Design: Andrea Meyer, emDASH inc.

Copyright © 1996
Chapman & Hall

Printed in the United States of America

For more information, contact:

Chapman & Hall	Chapman & Hall
115 Fifth Avenue	2-6 Boundary Row
New York, NY 10003	London SE1 8HN
	England

The products and/or brand names referred to in this manual are provided as a reference but do not reflect an endorsement of the product by the authors or publisher.

All rights reserved. No part of this work covered by the copyright hereon may be reproduced or used in any form or by any means—graphic, electronic, or mechanical, including photocopying, recording, taping, or information storage and retrieval systems —without the written permission of the publisher.

2 3 4 5 6 7 8 9 10 XXX 01 00 99 97

Library of Congress Cataloging-in-Publication Data

Pediatric nutrition handbook / Jil Feldhausen . . . [et al.].
    p.   cm. — (Chapman & Hall nutrition handbooks : 3)
    Includes bibliographical references.
    ISBN 0–412–07511–3
    1. Children—Nutrition—Handbooks, manual, etc. 2. Infants—Nutrition— Handbooks, manual, etc. I Feldhausen, Jil, 1956- . II. Series.
RM217.2.C44 1996 vol. 3
[RJ206}
615.8'54 s—dc20
[613.2'083]   95–19197
                                                                                        CIP

British Library Cataloguing in Publication Data available

To order this or any other Chapman & Hall book, please contact **International Thomson Publishing, 7625 Empire Drive, Florence, KY 41042. Phone: (606) 525-6600. Fax: (606) 525-7778, e-mail: order@chaphall.com.**

For a complete listing of Chapman & Hall's titles, send your requests to **Chapman & Hall, Dept. BC, 115 Fifth Avenue, New York, NY 10003.**

Preface

More than ever, health care practitioners are expected to provide nutritional care and guidance for their patients. The role of nutrition in disease prevention, health promotion, and therapeutics continues to expand and is of particular importance to the normal growth and development of infants and children.

This handbook was developed by a team of health care practitioners in nutrition and pediatrics. Its purpose is to provide clinicians with the essential knowledge to provide optimal nutritional care for pediatric patients. This handbook provides the necessary information to quickly and effectively assess nutritional status, develop an individual nutritional care plan, and provide dietary and nutritional guidance.

Great thanks goes to Julia Meyer, Class of 1996, who with wonderful humor and great patience helped bring this manual to a readable form from the perspective of a medical student. We would also like to express our gratitude to Kathleen Jaegers for her thoroughness and word processing expertise in the design and development of this handbook. Thanks also to Tina Leonard-Green for her editorial support and Chris Tisch for her typing assistance.

This handbook was made possible through NIH/NCI Grant No. CA-53459, Nutrition Education Curriculum for the Medical School.

It is our hope that this manual will be a valuable tool for providing care to pediatric patients.

Jil Feldhausen, MS, RD
  Clinical Lecturer
Doug Taren, PhD
  Principal Investigator, Nutrition Curriculum
  in Medical Education
Cynthia Thomson MS, RD
  Coordinator, Nutrition Curriculum
Department of Family and Community Medicine
Burris Duncan, MD
  Professor
  Department of Pediatrics
University of Arizona, Tucson

Table of Contents

	Page
PREFACE	v
LIST OF TABLES AND FIGURES	viii
ABBREVIATION	xvii

SECTION 1 GENERAL NUTRITION	1
NUTRITIONAL ASSESSMENT AT WELL-CHILD CHECKUPS	1
T.1.1 Nutritional Assessment and Counseling Guidelines	*2*
RECOMMENDED DIETARY ALLOWANCES	1
T.1.2 Recommended Dietary Allowances	*7*
RECOMMENDATIONS FOR VITAMIN/MINERAL SUPPLEMENTATION	1
T.1.3 Vitamin/Mineral Supplement Guide	*11*
FOOD GUIDE PYRAMID	15
F.1.1 Food Guide Pyramid	*15*
RECOMMENDED FOOD INTAKE	16
Birth to 2 Years of Age	16
T.1.4 Feeding Guidelines: Birth to 2 Years of Age	*17*
2 to 4 Years of Age	16
T.1.5 Feeding Guidelines: 2 to 4 Years of Age	*20*
5 to 18 Years of Age	16
T.1.6 Feeding Guidelines: 5 to 18 Years of Age	*21*

SECTION 2 FOOD SOURCES OF SELECTED NUTRIENTS	22
DIETARY SOURCES OF NUTRIENTS	22
T.2.1 Calcium	*22*
T.2.2 Fiber	*23*
T.2.3 Iron	*24*
T.2.4 Potassium	*25*
T.2.5 Sodium	*26*

T.2.6	*Vitamin A*	27
T.2.7	*Vitamin C*	27
T.2.8	*Vitamin D*	28
T.2.9	*Vitamin E*	28

ENERGY AND PROTEIN CONTENT OF SELECTED FOODS 29

T.2.10	*Energy and Protein Content of Selected Common Foods*	29
T.2.11	*Energy and Protein Content of Selected Baby Foods*	30
T.2.12	*Energy Concentrations of Standard Infant Foods*	31

SECTION 3   DETERMINATION OF NUTRIENT REQUIREMENTS 32

RECOMMENDATIONS FOR FLUID, ENERGY, AND PROTEIN 32

T.3.1	*Calculating Fluid Requirements*	32
T.3.2	*Calculating Energy Requirements*	33
T.3.3	*Calculating Protein Requirements*	34
T.3.4	*Quantity of Formula Required to Meet Energy Needs*	34

SECTION 4   ASSESSMENT OF NUTRITIONAL STATUS   35

FACTORS ASSOCIATED WITH NUTRITIONAL RISK IN CHILDREN 35

NUTRITIONAL STATUS ASSESSMENT 36

T.4.1	*Key Components of the Nutritional Status Assessment*	37
F.4.1	*Nutrition Status Assessment Form*	38

EVALUATING GROWTH 39

Average Weight Gain 40

T.4.2	*Average Weight Gain*	40

Growth Charts 41

F.4.2	*Girls' Growth: Birth to 36 Months of Age*	42
F.4.3	*Girls' Weight for Length: Birth to 36 Months of Age*	43
F.4.4	*Boys' Growth: Birth to 36 Months of Age*	44
F.4.5	*Boys' Weight for Length: Birth to 36 Months of Age*	45

F.4.6	*Girls' Growth: 2 to 18 Years of Age*	46
F.4.7	*Girls' Weight for Height: 2 to 12 Years of Age*	47
F.4.8	*Boys' Growth: 2 to 18 Years of Age*	48
F.4.9	*Boys' Weight for Height: 2 to 12 Years of Age*	49

Other Methods to Measure Growth 50
    F.4.10 Techniques of Anthropometric Measurements 50
    T.4.3 Percentiles for Triceps Skinfolds 51
Assessment of Inadequate Growth: "Failure to Thrive" 53
  Definition of Failure to Thrive 53
  Causes of Failure to Thrive 53
  Severity Classifications of Failure to Thrive 54
    T.4.4 Calculating Percent of Standard 54
    T.4.5 Waterlow Classification Chart 54
Assessment of Excessive Fat Stores: "Obesity" 55
  Definition of Obesity 55
  Assessment of Obesity 55
    T.4.6 Body Fat Assessment Methods 56
Estimation of Normal Height and Weight 55
LABORATORY ASSESSMENT OF NUTRITIONAL STATUS 55
    T.4.7 Evaluation of Anemia 57
    T.4.8 Calcium Abnormalities 60
    T.4.9 Carbohydrate Abnormalities 61
    T.4.10 Lipid Assessment 62
    T.4.11 Protein Malnutrition 63
    T.4.12 Other Evaluations of Nutritional Status 64

SECTION 5   REFERRAL CRITERIA 65
NUTRITIONAL REFERRAL 65
  Indicators for Nutrition Referral 65
  Writing Nutrition Referrals/Consults 66
    Sample Referrals 66
SUPPLEMENTAL FEEDING PROGRAMS FOR WOMEN, INFANTS, AND CHILDREN 66
    T.5.1 Summary of Two Supplemental Feeding Programs 67
  Other Referral Agencies 66

x Table of Contents

SECTION 6   AGE-SPECIFIC RECOMMENDATIONS
68

FEEDING INFANTS 68
Breastfeeding Basics 68
Algorithm for Successful Breastfeeding 68
    F.6.1   Algorithm for
          Successful Breastfeeding 69
Advantages of Breastfeeding 68
Weight Gain Velocity for Breastfed Infants 70
Breastmilk Storage 70
    T.6.1   Safe Storage Times for Breastmilk 70
Recommendations for Working Mothers 71
How to Respond to Concerns of
Lactating Women 71
    T.6.2   Breastfeeding Tips 72
    T.6.3   Possible Problematic Medications
          During Lactation 78
    T.6.4   Foods and Beverages Which May
          Cause G.I. Distress to Breastfeeding
          Infants 78
Breastfeeding Resources 79
Infant Formulas 79
    Formulas and Methods of Preparation 79
    T.6.5   Types of Formulas and Methods
          of Preparation 80
    Selection and Composition of Commercial
    Infant Formulas 79
    T.6.6   Composition of Milk-Based Formulas ... 81
    T.6.7   Composition of Soy-Based Formulas 82
    T.6.8   Composition of Special Use
          Infant Formulas 83
Altering Energy Intake 84
    T.6.9   Increasing Energy Intake for Weight
          Gain in Infants 84
    T.6.10   Altering Energy Concentrations of
           Liquid Formulas 84
    T.6.11   Altering Energy Concentrations of
           Powdered Formulas 85
    T.6.12   Increasing Energy Concentrations of
           Infant Formulas 85
Introducing Solid Foods 86
    Guidelines for Introducing Solid Foods 86
    T.6.13   Steps for Introducing Solid Foods 86

Guidelines to Reduce Risk of Choking 87
Making Eating Safer for Young Children 87
   T.6.14 *Foods That Can Cause Choking in*
           Children Until Age 5 87
   T.6.15 *Foods **Not** to Feed to Infants* 89
Promoting Healthy Teeth 88
Teething Tips 88
Proper Bottle Use Advice 88
   T.6.16 *Teeth and Gum Care Guidelines* 90
FEEDING TODDLERS AND YOUNG CHILDREN 88
Increasing Energy Intake for Young Children 90
   T.6.17 *Increasing Energy Intake for Weight*
           Gain in Young Children 91
   T.6.18 *Feeding Solutions* 92
   T.6.19 *Ideas for Balanced Meals*
           and Snacks 94
   T.6.20 *Nutritious Snacks* 97
FEEDING SCHOOL-AGE AND
ADOLESCENT CHILDREN 98
Dietary Fat 98
   T.6.21 *Reducing Fat Intake in School-Age*
           and Adolescent Children 98
Factors Associated with Nutritional Risk 99
Importance of Breakfast/School Feeding 99
   F.6.2 *Food in the Morning: "Food*
          for Excellence" 100
Sports Nutrition 99
   What Should Athletes Eat? 99
   Weight Control 99
   Pregame Meals 99
   Eating for All-Day Sporting Events 101
   Convenient Snacks for the Athlete 101
   Water Requirements 101
   Vitamin/Mineral Supplementation 102

SECTION 7   DISEASE-SPECIFIC FEEDING ISSUES 103
   T.7.1 *Common Diet-Related Problems* 104
CARDIOVASCULAR DISEASE 106
Screening Recommendations 106
   T.7.2 *Evaluation of Serum*
          Cholesterol Levels 106

Table of Contents

      T.7.3 Current vs. Recommended Fat Intake in Children and Adolescents with CVD . 106
  Dietary Intervention for the Prevention and Treatment of Cardiovascular Disease 107
      T.7.4 Recommended Intakes on the Step-One and Step-Two Diets 107
      T.7.5 Diet Therapy vs. Drug Therapy in CVD Treatment 108
EATING DISORDERS 109
  General Information 109
  Suggestions Which May Help Reduce Risk of Developing an Eating Disorder 109
  Recommended Treatment/Intervention for Eating Disorders 109
  Anorexia Nervosa 110
    Signs to Look For 110
    Nutritional Therapy 110
      T.7.6 Healthy Eating Patterns in Anorexia Nervosa 111
  Bulimia Nervosa 111
    Signs to Look For 111
    Nutritional Therapy 111
      T.7.7 Mifflin Resting Energy Expenditure Formulas 112
      T.7.8 Healthy Eating Patterns in Bulimia Nervosa 112
OBESITY 113
  Nature Versus Nurture 113
  Treatment for Obesity 113
      T.7.9 Guidelines for Reducing Energy and Fat Intake 114
      T.7.10 Ideas for Increasing Energy Expenditure 115
FOOD ALLERGIES 115
      T.7.11 Egg-Free Diet 116
      T.7.12 Milk-Free Diet 118
      T.7.13 Wheat-Free Diet 121

REFERENCES & SUGGESTED READINGS 123

INDEX 125

List of Tables and Figures

		Page
SECTION 1	GENERAL NUTRITION	
Table 1.1	Nutritional Assessment and Counseling Guidelines	2
Figure 1.1	Food Guide Pyramid	15
Table 1.2	Recommended Dietary Allowances	7
Table 1.3	Vitamin/Mineral Supplement Guide	11
Table 1.4	Feeding Guidelines: Birth to 2 Years of Age	17
Table 1.5	Feeding Guidelines: 2 to 4 Years of Age	20
Table 1.6	Feeding Guidelines: 5 to 18 Years of Age	21
SECTION 2	FOOD SOURCES OF SELECTED NUTRIENTS	
Table 2.1	Dietary Sources of Calcium	22
Table 2.2	Dietary Sources of Fiber	23
Table 2.3	Dietary Sources of Iron	24
Table 2.4	Dietary Sources of Potassium	25
Table 2.5	Dietary Sources of Sodium	26
Table 2.6	Dietary Sources of Vitamin A	27
Table 2.7	Dietary Sources of Vitamin C	27
Table 2.8	Dietary Sources of Vitamin D	28
Table 2.9	Dietary Sources of Vitamin E	28
Table 2.10	Energy and Protein Content of Selected Common Foods	29
Table 2.11	Energy and Protein Content of Selected Baby Foods	30
Table 2.12	Energy Concentrations of Standard Infant Foods	31
SECTION 3	DETERMINATION OF NUTRIENT REQUIREMENTS	
Table 3.1	Calculating Fluid Requirements	32
Table 3.2	Calculating Energy Requirements	33
Table 3.3	Calculating Protein Requirements	34

Table 3.4	Quantity of Formula Required to Meet Energy Needs	34
SECTION 4	**ASSESSMENT OF NUTRITIONAL STATUS**	
Figure 4.1	Nutrition Status Assessment Form	38
Table 4.1	Key Components of the Nutritional Status Assessment	37
Table 4.2	Average Weight Gain	40
Figure 4.2	Girls' Growth: Birth to 36 Months of Age	42
Figure 4.3	Girls' Weight for Length: Birth to 36 Months of Age	43
Figure 4.4	Boys' Growth: Birth to 36 Months of Age	44
Figure 4.5	Boys' Weight for Length: Birth to 36 Months of Age	45
Figure 4.6	Girls' Growth: 2 to 18 Years of Age	46
Figure 4.7	Girls' Weight for Height: 2 to 12 Years of Age	47
Figure 4.8	Boys' Growth: 2 to 18 Years of Age	48
Figure 4.9	Boys' Weight for Height: 2 to 12 Years of Age	49
Figure 4.10	Techniques of Anthropometric Measurements	50
Table 4.3	Percentiles for Triceps Skinfolds for Whites of the U.S.	51
Table 4.4	Calculating Percent of Standard Weight for Height	54
Table 4.5	Waterlow Classification Chart	54
Table 4.6	Body Fat Assessment Methods	56
Table 4.7	Evaluation of Anemia	57
Table 4.8	Calcium Abnormalities	60
Table 4.9	Carbohydrate Abnormalities	61
Table 4.10	Lipid Assessment	62
Table 4.11	Protein Malnutrition	63
Table 4.12	Other Evaluations of Nutritional Status	64
SECTION 5	**REFERRAL CRITERIA**	
Table 5.1	Summary of Two Supplemental Feeding Programs	67
SECTION 6	**AGE-SPECIFIC RECOMMENDATIONS**	
Figure 6.1	Algorithm for Successful Breastfeeding	69
Table 6.1	Safe Storage Times for Breastmilk	70

Table 6.2	Breastfeeding Tips	72
Table 6.3	Possible Problematic Medications During Lactation	78
Table 6.4	Foods and Beverages Which May Cause G.I. Distress to Breastfeeding Infants	78
Table 6.5	Types of Formulas and Methods of Preparation	80
Table 6.6	Composition of Milk-Based Formulas	81
Table 6.7	Composition of Soy-Based Formulas	82
Table 6.8	Composition of Special Use Infant Formulas	83
Table 6.9	Increasing Energy Intake for Weight Gain in Infants	84
Table 6.10	Altering Energy Concentrations of Liquid Formulas	84
Table 6.11	Altering Energy Concentrations of Powdered Formulas	85
Table 6.12	Increasing Energy Concentrations of Infant Formulas	85
Table 6.13	Steps for Introducing Solid Foods	86
Table 6.14	Foods That Can Cause Choking in Children Until Age 5	87
Table 6.15	Foods *Not* to Feed to Infants	89
Table 6.16	Teeth and Gum Care Guidelines	90
Table 6.17	Increasing Energy Intake for Weight Gain in Young Children	91
Table 6.18	Childhood Feeding Problems and Solutions	92
Table 6.19	Ideas for Balanced Meals and Snacks	94
Table 6.20	Healthy Snacks for Young Children	97
Table 6.21	Reducing Fat Intake in School-Age and Adolescent Children	98
Figure 6.2	Food in the Morning: "Food for Excellence"	100
SECTION 7	DISEASE-SPECIFIC FEEDING ISSUES	
Table 7.1	Common Diet-Related Problems	104
Table 7.2	Evaluation of Serum Cholesterol Levels	106
Table 7.3	Current vs. Recommended Fat Intake in Children and Adolescents with CVD	106
Table 7.4	Recommended Intakes on the Step-One and Step-Two Diets	107

Table 7.5	Diet Therapy vs. Drug Therapy in CVD Treatment	108
Table 7.6	Healthy Eating Patterns in Anorexia Nervosa	111
Table 7.7	Mifflin Resting Energy Expenditure Formulas	112
Table 7.8	Healthy Eating Patterns in Bulimia Nervosa	112
Table 7.9	Guidelines for Reducing Energy and Fat Intake	114
Table 7.10	Ideas for Increasing Energy Expenditure	115
Table 7.11	Egg-Free Diet	116
Table 7.12	Milk-Free Diet	118
Table 7.13	Wheat-Free Diet	121

Abbreviations

BMI	body mass index
cc	cubic centimeter (liquid measurement)
cm	centimeter
CVD	cardiovascular disease
Diet Rx	diet prescription
dL	deciliter
°F	degrees Fahrenheit
Fe^+	iron
$FeSO_4$	iron sulfate
fl oz	fluid ounce
G.I.	gastrointestinal
gm	gram
H_2	hydrogen
HC	head circumference
Hct	hematocrit
HDL	high density lipoprotein
Hgb	hemoglobin
H/H	hemoglobin/hematocrit
ht	height
IgA	immunoglobulin A
IgE	immunoglobulin E
in.	inch
IU	international unit
kcal	kilocalorie
kg	kilogram
/L	per liter
lb	pound
LDL	low density lipoprotein
MAC	mid-arm circumference
MAMC	mid-arm muscle circumference
MCHC	mean corpuscular hemoglobin concentration
MCT	medium chain triglycerides
MCV	mean corpuscular volume
mEq	milliequivalent
mg	milligram
min	minute
ml	milliliter

mmol	millimole
mos.	months
NCHS	National Center for Health Statistics
ng	nanogram
NSA	Nutrition Status Assessment
oz	ounce
%tile	percentile
ppm	parts per million
RBC	red blood cell
RDA	Recommended Dietary Allowances
REE	resting energy expenditure
svg	serving
Tbsp	tablespoon
TIBC	total iron binding capacity
TSF	triceps skinfolds
tsp	teaspoon
UBW	usual body weight
USDA	United States Department of Agriculture
WIC	Women, Infants, and Children
wk	week
wt	weight
y/o	years old
µg	microgram

SECTION 1
General Nutrition

Nutritional Assessment at Well-Child Checkups

Nutritional care is an essential component of pediatric medical care. Table 1.1 is designed to facilitate the incorporation of nutritional assessment at each well check, making this also an excellent opportunity to offer nutritional guidance. Parents usually have many questions regarding eating behavior, developmental changes, and diet adequacy during this period of rapid growth. Table 1.1 includes guidelines for nutritional assessment, including dietary history, anthropometric measurements (height and weight), and laboratory evaluation. The column on counseling/handouts provides suggested topics for discussion at each patient visit. Children's developmental needs will vary, and some topics such as dietary adequacy should be covered in most visits.

Recommended Dietary Allowances

"Recommended Dietary Allowances (RDA) are the levels of intake of essential nutrients considered in the judgment of the Committee on Dietary Allowances of the Food and Nutrition Board, on the basis of available scientific knowledge, to be adequate to meet or exceed known nutritional needs of practically all *healthy persons*."

RDAs (see Table 1.2, pgs 7 to 10) reflect the average daily intakes which populations should consume over time and are not individual requirements.

Recommendations for Vitamin/Mineral Supplementation

Table 1.3 (pgs 11 to 14), the ***Vitamin/Mineral Supplement Guide***, identifies the nutrients for which the RDA may be difficult to meet in infancy and/or childhood.

Table 1.1
NUTRITIONAL ASSESSMENT AND COUNSELING GUIDELINES

Age	Assessment	Counseling/Handouts
2 weeks	• Breastfeeding issues. • Formula iron-fortification and preparation techniques. • History for colic. • Measure and plot height (ht), weight (wt), and head circumference (HC) on the National Center for Health Statistics (NCHS) graph (Figures 4.2, 4.3, 4.4, and 4.5).	• Provide information and answers to breastfeeding issues (Tables 6.1–6.4). • Feed baby on demand; hold baby in arms for feeding. • If breastfeeding, mother should continue taking prenatal vitamins/minerals and consume an adequate diet. • Breastfeeding babies should be given 0.25 mg/day fluoride supplement (Table 1.3). • Formula-fed babies may need extra water when ambient temperature increases. • If infant's weight gain is inadequate (based on plotted ht, wt, and HC) (Tables 3.2, 3.3, 3.4, 4.4, 4.5, 6.9, 6.10, 6.11, and 6.12).
2 months	• Diet history, checking for feeding frequency; no progression to solid foods. • Measure and plot ht, wt, and HC on NCHS graph (Figures 4.2, 4.3, 4.4, and 4.5).	• Breastfeeding babies should be given 0.25 mg/day fluoride supplement (Table 1.3). • Breastmilk and iron-fortified formula are adequate for infant's nutritional needs. • No solids until 4–6 months of age. • No cereal in bottles. • If infant's weight gain is inadequate (based on plotted ht, wt, and HC) (Tables 3.2, 3.3, 3.4, 4.4, 4.5, 6.9, 6.10, 6.11, and 6.12).

Table 1.1
NUTRITIONAL ASSESSMENT AND COUNSELING GUIDELINES *Continued*

Age	Assessment	Counseling/Handouts
4 months	• Diet history, checking for readiness for solid foods. • Measure and plot ht, wt, and HC on NCHS graph (Figures 4.2, 4.3, 4.4, and 4.5).	• Provide infant source of iron (formula, cereal, or supplement) (Table 2.3). • See *Recommended Food Intake* (Table 1.4). • See *Introducing Solid Foods* (Table 6.13). • See *Vitamin/Mineral Supplement Guide* (Table 1.3). • If infant's weight gain is inadequate (based on plotted ht, wt, and HC) (Tables 3.2, 3.3, 3.4, 4.4, 4.5, 6.9, 6.10, 6.11, and 6.12).
6 months	• Diet history, checking for introduction of solid foods. • Measure and plot ht, wt, and HC on NCHS graph (Figures 4.2, 4.3, 4.4, and 4.5). • Evaluate iron intake and anemia.	• Never leave baby alone when eating (Table 6.14). • See *Recommended Food Intake* (Table 1.4). • See *Introducing Solid Foods* (Table 6.13). • See *Foods NOT to Feed Infants* (Table 6.15). • See *Vitamin/Mineral Supplement Guide* (Table 1.3). • See *Dietary Sources of Iron* (Table 2.3). • See *Anemia* (Table 4.7). • Delay cow's milk until 1 y/o due to renal solute load high; iron and vitamin C low. • If infant's weight gain is inadequate (based on plotted ht, wt, and HC) (Tables 3.2, 3.3, 3.4, 4.4, 4.5, 6.9, 6.10, 6.11, and 6.12).

continued on next page

Table 1.1
NUTRITIONAL ASSESSMENT AND COUNSELING GUIDELINES Continued

Age	Assessment	Counseling/Handouts
9–12 months	• Diet history, checking for type and quantity of milk, presence of solid foods. • Evaluate for calcium, iron, vitamin A, and vitamin C intake. • Measure and plot ht, wt, and HC on NCHS graph (Figures 4.2, 4.3, 4.4, and 4.5).	• Formula or milk intake should be less than 32 oz (Table 3.1). • No bottles in bed. • See *Recommended Food Intake* (Table 1.4). • See *Introducing Solid Foods* (Table 6.13). • See *Dietary Sources of Calcium, Iron, Vitamin A, and Vitamin C* (Section 2). • Change to cow's milk (possible constipation). • If infant's weight gain is inadequate (based on plotted ht, wt, and HC) (Tables 3.2, 3.3, 3.4, 4.4, 4.5, 6.9, 6.10, 6.11, and 6.12).
15 months	• Diet history, checking for progression to table foods. • Measure and plot ht, wt, and HC on NCHS graph (Figures 4.2, 4.3, 4.4, and 4.5).	• Provide a variety of foods, and allow child to choose quantities. • Feed child table foods at meals with family. • See *Recommended Food Intake* (Table 1.4). • See *Ideas for Balanced Meals and Snacks* (Table 6.19). • See *Nutritious Snacks* (Table 6.20). • If child's weight gain is inadequate (based on plotted ht, wt, and HC) (Tables 4.4, 4.5, 6.17, 6.18 and 6.20).

Table 1.1
NUTRITIONAL ASSESSMENT AND COUNSELING GUIDELINES *Continued*

Age	Assessment	Counseling/Handouts
18 months	• Diet history, nutritious snacks. • Measure and plot ht, wt, and HC on NCHS graph (Figures 4.2, 4.3, 4.4, and 4.5).	• Three meals and 2-3 snacks should be provided consistently to child. • See *Recommended Food Intake* (Table 1.4). • See *Nutritious Snacks* (Table 6.20). • See *Ideas for Balanced Meals and Snacks* (Table 6.19). • See *Feeding Solutions* (Table 6.18). • If child's weight gain is inadequate (based on plotted ht, wt, and HC) (Tables 4.4, 4.5, 6.17, 6.18 and 6.20).
24 months	• Diet history, nutritious snacks. • Measure and plot ht, wt, and HC on NCHS graph (Figures 4.2, 4.3, 4.4, and 4.5).	• Avoid battles over food. • Food should not be used as a reward See *Feeding Solutions* (Table 6.18). • See *Recommended Food Intake* (Table 1.5). • See *Nutritious Snacks* (Table 6.20). • See *Ideas for Balanced Meals and Snacks* (Table 6.19). • If child's weight gain is inadequate (based on plotted ht, wt, and HC) (Tables 4.4, 4.5, 6.17, 6.18 and 6.20).

continued on next page

Table 1.1
NUTRITIONAL ASSESSMENT AND COUNSELING GUIDELINES *Continued*

Age	Assessment	Counseling/Handouts
3–10 years	• Diet history, checking for balanced diet. • Measure and plot ht, wt, and HC on NCHS graph (Figures 4.6, 4.7, 4.8, and 4.9). • Evaluate activity level. • Evaluate blood pressure. • Evaluate cholesterol.	• Encourage healthy eating and activity habits (Tables 6.19, 6.20, 6.21, and 7.9). • See *Recommended Food Intake* (Tables 1.5 and 1.6). • See *Healthy Snacks* (Table 6.20). • See *Ideas for Balanced Meals and Snacks* (Table 6.19). • See *Food in the Morning* (Figure 6.2) If child's weight gain is inadequate (based on plotted ht, wt, and HC) (Tables 4.4, 4.5, 6.17, 6.18 and 6.20).
11–18 years	• Diet history, checking for balanced diet. • Measure and plot ht, wt, and HC on NCHS graph (Figures 4.6, 4.7, 4.8, and 4.9). • Evaluate activity level. • Evaluate anemia. • Evaluate blood pressure. • Evaluate cholesterol.	• Encourage healthy eating and activity habits (Table 6.20, 6.21 and 7.9). • See *Recommended Food Intake* (Table 1.6). • See *Sports Nutrition* (Section 6). • See *Eating Disorders* (Section 7). • See *Evaluation of Serum Cholesterol* (Table 7.2). • See *Evaluation of Uremia* (Table 4.9). • See *Food in the Morning* (Figure 6.2).

Table 1.2
RECOMMENDED DIETARY ALLOWANCES

Category	Age (years)	Weight[b] (kg)	Weight[b] (lb)	Height[b] (cm)	Height[b] (in)	Protein (gm)	Vitamin A (μg RE)[c]	Fat-Soluble Vitamins Vitamin D (μg)[d]	Vitamin E (mg α-TE)[e]	Vitamin K (μg)
Infants	0.0–0.5	6	13	60	24	13	375	7.5	3	5
	0.5–1.0	9	20	71	28	14	375	10	4	10
Children	1–3	13	29	90	35	16	400	10	6	15
	4–6	20	44	112	44	24	500	10	7	20
	7–10	28	62	132	52	28	700	10	7	30
Males	11–14	45	99	157	62	45	1,000	10	10	45
	15–18	66	145	176	69	59	1,000	10	10	65
	19–24	72	160	177	70	58	1,000	10	10	70
	25–50	79	174	176	70	63	1,000	5	10	80
	51+	77	170	173	68	63	1,000	5	10	80
Females	11–14	46	101	157	62	46	800	10	8	45
	15–18	55	120	163	64	44	800	10	8	55
	19–24	58	128	164	65	46	800	10	8	60
	25–50	63	138	163	64	50	800	5	8	65
	51+	65	143	160	63	50	800	5	8	65
Pregnant						60	800	10	10	65
Lactating 1st 6 months						65	1,300	10	12	65
2nd 6 months						62	1,200	10	11	65

continued on next page

Table 1.2
RECOMMENDED DIETARY ALLOWANCES *Continued*

Category	Age (years)	Weight[b] (kg)	Weight[b] (lb)	Height[b] (cm)	Height[b] (in)	Protein (gm)	Vitamin C (mg)	Thiamine (mg)	Riboflavin (mg)	Niacin (mg NE)	Vitamin B_6 (mg)	Folate (µg)	Vitamin B_{12} (µg)
Infants	0.0–0.5	6	13	60	24	13	30	0.3	0.4	5	0.3	25	0.3
	0.5–1.0	9	20	71	28	14	35	0.4	0.5	6	0.6	35	0.5
Children	1–3	13	29	90	35	16	40	0.7	0.8	9	1.0	50	0.7
	4–6	20	44	112	44	24	45	0.9	1.1	12	1.1	75	1.0
	7–10	28	62	132	52	28	45	1.0	1.2	13	1.4	100	1.4
Males	11–14	45	99	157	62	45	50	1.3	1.5	17	1.7	150	2.0
	15–18	66	145	176	69	59	60	1.5	1.8	20	2.0	200	2.0
	19–24	72	160	177	70	58	60	1.5	1.7	19	2.0	200	2.0
	25–50	79	174	176	70	63	60	1.5	1.7	19	2.0	200	2.0
	51+	77	170	173	68	63	60	1.2	1.4	15	2.0	200	2.0
Females	11–14	46	101	157	62	46	50	1.1	1.3	15	1.4	150	2.0
	15–18	55	120	163	64	44	60	1.1	1.3	15	1.5	180	2.0
	19–24	58	128	164	65	46	60	1.1	1.3	15	1.6	180	2.0
	25–50	63	138	163	64	50	60	1.1	1.3	15	1.6	180	2.0
	51+	65	143	160	63	50	60	1.0	1.2	13	1.6	180	2.0
Pregnant						60	70	1.5	1.6	17	2.2	400	2.2
Lactating 1st 6 months						65	95	1.6	1.8	20	2.1	280	2.6
2nd 6 months						62	90	1.6	1.7	20	2.1	260	2.6

Table 1.2
RECOMMENDED DIETARY ALLOWANCES *Continued*

Category	Age (years)	Weight[b] (kg)	Weight[b] (lb)	Height[b] (cm)	Height[b] (in)	Protein (gm)	Minerals Calcium (mg)	Phosphorus (mg)	Magnesium (mg)	Iron (mg)	Zinc (mg)	Iodine (µg)	Selenium (µg)
Infants	0.0–0.5	6	13	60	24	13	400	300	40	6	5	40	10
	0.5–1.0	9	20	71	28	14	600	500	60	10	5	50	15
Children	1–3	13	29	90	35	16	800	800	80	10	10	70	20
	4–6	20	44	112	44	24	800	800	120	10	10	90	20
	7–10	28	62	132	52	28	800	800	170	10	10	120	30
Males	11–14	45	99	157	62	45	1,200	1,200	270	12	15	150	40
	15–18	66	145	176	69	59	1,200	1,200	400	12	15	150	50
	19–24	72	160	177	70	58	1,200	1,200	350	10	15	150	70
	25–50	79	174	176	70	63	800	800	350	10	15	150	70
	51+	77	170	173	68	63	800	800	350	10	15	150	70
Females	11–14	46	101	157	62	46	1,200	1,200	280	15	12	150	45
	15–18	55	120	163	64	44	1,200	1,200	300	15	12	150	50
	19–24	58	128	164	65	46	1,200	1,200	280	15	12	150	55
	25–50	63	138	163	64	50	800	800	280	15	12	150	55
	51+	65	143	160	63	50	800	800	280	10	12	150	55
Pregnant						60	1,200	1,200	320	30	15	175	65
Lactating 1st 6 months						65	1,200	1,200	355	15	19	200	75
2nd 6 months						62	1,200	1,200	340	15	16	200	75

continued on next page

Table 1.2
RECOMMENDED DIETARY ALLOWANCES *Continued*

[a] The allowances, expressed as average daily intakes over time, are intended to provide for individual variations among most normal persons as they live in the United States under usual environmental stresses. Diets should be based on a variety of common foods in order to provide other nutrients for which human requirements have been less well defined.

[b] Weights and heights of Reference Adults are actual medians for the US population of the designated age, as reported by NHANES II. The use of these figures does not imply that the height-to-weight ratios are ideal.

[c] Retinol equivalents. 1 retinol equivalent = 1 µg retinol or 6 µg β-carotene.

[d] As cholecalciferol. 10 µg cholecalciferol = 400 IU of vitamin D.

[e] α-Tocopherol equivalents. 1 mg d-α tocopherol = 1 α-TE.

Reprinted with permission from Recommended Dietary Allowances, 10th ed. Copyright 1989 by the National Academy of Sciences. Courtesy of the National Academy Press, Washington, DC.

Table 1.3
VITAMIN/MINERAL SUPPLEMENT GUIDE

Vitamin/ Mineral	Age (yrs)	RDAs		Supplementation Recommendations
Vitamin A		μg	IU	
	Preemie	375	(1875)	• Breastmilk and formula are adequate.
	0–0.5	375	(1875)	• "
	0.5–1	375	(1875)	• "
	1–3	400	(2000)	• No supplement recommended (see *Vitamin A Sources*, Table 2.6).
	4–6	500	(2500)	• "
	7–10	700	(3500)	• "
	11–14 males	1000	(5000)	• "
	11–14 females	800	(4000)	• "
	15–18 males	1000	(5000)	• "
	15–18 females	800	(4000)	• "
Vitamin C		mg		
	Preemie	30		• Controversial. Use preterm formula and human milk fortifier.
	0–0.5	30		• Breastmilk and formula are adequate.
	0.5–1	35		• Eat fruits and vegetables (see *Vitamin C Sources*, Table 2.7).
	1–3	40		• "
	4–6	45		• "
	7–10	45		• "
	11–14	50		• "
	15–18	60		• "

continued on next page

Table 1.3
VITAMIN/MINERAL SUPPLEMENT GUIDE *Continued*

Vitamin/ Mineral	Age (yrs)	RDAs		Supplementation Recommendations
Vitamin D		µg	IU	
	Preemie	12.5	(500)	• Supplement with 12.5 µg until 2.5 kg.
	0–0.5	7.5	(300)	• Supplement with 5–7.5 µg if no sunshine exposure or dark pigmentation and exclusively breastfed.
	0.5–1	10	(400)	• Supplement with 10 µg if no sunshine exposure or dark pigmentation and exclusively breastfed.
	1–3	10	(400)	• Drink fortified milk (see *Vitamin D Sources*, Table 2.8).
	4–6	10	(400)	• "
	7–10	10	(400)	• "
	11–14 males	10	(400)	• "
	11–14 females	10	(400)	• "
	15–18 males	10	(400)	• "
	15–18 females	10	(400)	• "
Vitamin E		mg	IU	
	Preemie	5–25		• Supplement with 5–25 IU (mg).
	0–0.5	3	(3)	• Breastmilk and formula are adequate.
	0.5–1	4	(4)	• Breastmilk and formula are adequate.
	1–3	6	(6)	• Eat a varied diet (see *Vitamin E Sources*, Table 2.9).
	4–6	7	(7)	• "
	7–10	7	(7)	• "
	11–14 males	10	(10)	• "
	11–14 females	8	(8)	• "
	15–18 males	10	(10)	• "
	15–18 females	9	(8)	• "

TABLE 1.3
VITAMIN/MINERAL SUPPLEMENT GUIDE Continued

Vitamin/Mineral	Age (yrs)	RDAs	Supplementation Recommendations
Vitamin K	0–0.5	μg 5	• Newborn intramuscular injection (0.5-1 mg).
	0.5–1	10	• No supplement necessary.
	1–3	15	• "
	4–6	20	• "
	7–10	30	• "
	11–14	45	• "
Calcium	0–0.5	mg 400	• Breastmilk and formula are adequate.
	0.5–1.0	600	• "
	1–3	800	• Consume dairy products or supplement (see *Calcium Sources*, Table 2.1).
	4–6	800	• "
	7–10	800	• "
	11–14	1200	• "
	15–18	1200	• "
Fluoride	0–2	mg/day* 0.25	• Breastfed infants require supplementation. *Formula-fed infants who use local water do not need additional fluorides.*
	2–3	0.25	• Dependent on local water.*
	3–16	0.50	• Dependent on local water.*

* *Contact local water department for fluoride levels. If fluoride content of water is <0.3 ppm, fluoride supplementation is recommended by the American Academy of Pediatrics.*

continued on next page

Table 1.3
VITAMIN/MINERAL SUPPLEMENT GUIDE Continued

Vitamin/Mineral	Age (yrs)	RDAs	Supplementation Recommendations
Iron	Preemie	6	• Begin supplement at 2 kg. (If breastfed, supplement 2-3 mg/kg.* If formula-fed, use iron-fortified formula.)
	Term—4 months	10	• If breastfed, supplement at 4 months.** No supplement necessary with iron-fortified formula.
	4–12 months	10	• Eat iron-fortified cereal** or drink iron-fortified formula or provide iron supplement.
	1–10	10	• Monitor iron status (see Tables 2.3 and Table 4.7).
	11–18 males	12	"
	11–18 females	15	"
	15–18	65	• May need to supplement athlete (see Sports Nutrition, Section 6).

Source: "Nutritional Needs of Preterm Infants" in Pediatric Nutrition Handbook. Barnes LA (ed.) American Academy of Pediatrics. Elk Village, IL, 1993.

*Iron-fortified cereal has 1.77 mg iron/Tbsp.

Food Guide Pyramid

The Food Guide Pyramid was developed by the United States Department of Agriculture (USDA) in 1992 to provide Americans with a visual tool for healthy eating. The Pyramid (Figure 1.1) is based on scientific research of what Americans eat, what nutrients are in various foods, and how to make the best food choices for optimal health.

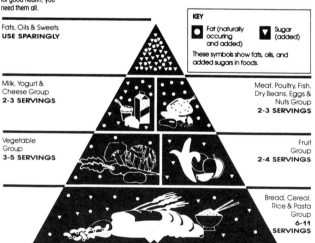

Figure 1.1
FOOD GUIDE PYRAMID

U.S. Department of Agriculture and the U.S. Department of Health and Human Resources, Food Guide Pyramid: A Guide to Daily Food Choices, *National Live Stock and Meat Board: Washington, DC, 1993.*

Recommended Food Intake

Birth to 2 Years of Age

Infants and very young children are emerging eaters. Servings increase in frequency and size. Initially, until 4-6 months of age, infants need only breastmilk or formula. Between 6-12 months of age, the types of food groups expand and by 1 year a child should be eating approximately 50% of his/her energy intake as solid food.

Table 1.4 represents a *guideline* of the average intake recommended for this age group. Many infants will eat more or less, depending on their energy needs. For example, an average intake for an 8-month-old infant would be four 8-oz servings of breastmilk or formula, two 4-Tbsp servings of baby cereal, three 4-Tbsp servings of baby fruits or vegetables, and a 3-oz serving of fruit juice.

2 to 4 Years of Age

Children need to eat small amounts of a variety of foods. Advise parents that children decide *how much* to eat and parents decide *what types of food to offer*. Children should never be forced to eat. Parents can best function as a role model by eating healthy foods. Table 1.5 is a guideline—not a specific recommendation—of what to offer children to provide a balanced diet.

5 to 18 Years of Age

Parents need to be encouraged to provide a variety of healthy, nutritious foods in sufficient quantity for growing children. Each child is born with a genetic blueprint for his height, weight, and growth pattern. Attempting to alter this is very risky, with little opportunity for positive outcome. The risk for developing behavior problems, food fights, and eating disorders are increased with too much parental interference. Parents are responsible for the types of foods purchased, available, and prepared for the home; children are responsible for what and how much they eat. The following tables provide guidelines—not specific recommendations—for feeding school-age and adolescent children.

Table 1.4
FEEDING GUIDELINES: BIRTH TO 2 YEARS OF AGE

Age (mos)	Food Group	Servings Per Day	Food Item	Serving Size
0–4	Milk	8–12 or on demand	Breastmilk	Varies
0–1	Milk	6–8	Formula	2–5 oz
1–2	Milk	5–7	Formula	3–6 oz
2–3	Milk	4–7	Formula	4–7 oz
3–4	Milk	4–7	Formula	6–8 oz
4–6	Milk Grain	4–6 or on demand 2	Breastmilk/Formula Baby cereal (iron-fortified)	6–8 oz 1–2 Tbsp
6–8	Milk Grain Fruits and Vegetables	3–5 or on demand 2 4	Breastmilk/Formula Baby cereal (iron-fortified) Bread, bagel, bun Crackers (no salt) Fruits, vegetables Baby fruit juice	6–8 oz 4 Tbsp 1/2 slice or 1/4 bagel 2 2–3 Tbsp 3 oz

Adapted from Airplanes, Choo-choos and Other Games Parents Play, National Dairy Council. Rosemont, etc. 1993.

continued on next page

Table 1.4
FEEDING GUIDELINES: BIRTH TO 2 YEARS OF AGE *Continued*

Age (mos)	Food Group	Servings Per Day	Food Item	Serving Size
8–12	Milk	3–4	Breastmilk/Formula, whole milk Cheese Yogurt (plain) Cottage cheese	6–8 oz 1/2 oz 1/2 cup 1/4 cup
	Grain	2	Baby cereal (iron-fortified) Bread, bagel Crackers (no salt)	2–4 Tbsp 1/2 slice or 1/4 bagel 2
	Fruits and Vegetables	4	Fruits, vegetables Baby fruit juice	3–4 Tbsp 3 oz
	Meat	2	Chicken, beef, pork Beans (cooked) Egg yolk (cooked)	3–4 Tbsp 1/2 cup 1

Adapted from Airplanes, Choo-choos and Other Games Parents Play, National Dairy Council. Rosemont, etc. 1993.

Table 1.4
FEEDING GUIDELINES: BIRTH TO 2 YEARS OF AGE *Continued*

Age (mos)	Food Group	Servings Per Day	Food Item	Serving Size
12–24	Milk	3	Whole milk, yogurt Cheese Cottage cheese	1/2 cup 1/2 oz 1/4 cup
	Grain	4	Cereal, pasta, rice Bread, muffin, bagel, roll Crackers	1/4 cup 1/4 cup 2
	Fruits and Vegetables	4	Fruit/vegetable (raw or cooked)	1/2 small or 1/4 cup
	Meat	2	Beef, chicken, fish, pork, turkey Bean or peas (cooked) Egg	1 oz 1/4 cup 1

Airplanes, Choo-choos and Other Games Parents Play, National Dairy Council. Rosemont, etc. 1993.

Table 1.5
FEEDING GUIDELINES: 2 TO 4 YEARS OF AGE

Food Groups	Servings Per Day	Serving Size
Fruits	2 or more svgs including at least 1 vitamin C source	1/2 small piece of fruit, such as apple, orange, or banana; 1/3 cup juice, 1/4 cup cooked fruit
Vegetables	3 or more svgs including at least 1 vitamin A source	1/2 cup leafy salad greens, 1/4 to 1/2 cup cooked vegetable, 1/2 cup raw vegetables
Grains	6 or more	1/2 oz ready-to-eat breakfast cereal; 1/2 slice whole grain bread; 1/4 cup cooked rice, pasta, or cereal; 4 crackers, 1/2 tortilla, muffin, or dinner roll; 1/4 bagel or hamburger bun
Milk, Cheese, Yogurt	2	1 cup low-fat or non-fat milk or yogurt; 1-1/2 oz cheese
Meat, Fish, Poultry, Beans, Eggs, and Nuts	2–3	1/2 oz cooked, lean meat, fish, or chicken. Substitute 1 egg; 1/4 cup cooked peas or beans; or 1 Tbsp peanut butter for 1/2 oz of meat
Fats, Oils, and Sweets	Go easy on these foods/beverages	Although dependent on size and age, fat recommendations are 43-60 gm/day or 30% of calories

Table 1.6
FEEDING GUIDELINES: 5 TO 18 YEARS OF AGE

Food Groups	Servings Per Day		Serving Size
	5–10 y/o	11–18 y/o	
Fruits	3 or more svgs including at least 1 vitamin C source	3 or more svgs including at least 1 vitamin C source	1 small piece of fruit, such as apple, orange, or banana, 1/2 cup juice, 1/2 cup cooked fruit
Vegetables	2 or more svgs including at least 1 vitamin A source	2 or more svgs including at least 1 vitamin A source	1 cup leafy salad greens, 1/2 cup cooked vegetables
Grains	6 or more	6 or more	1 oz ready-to-eat breakfast cereal; 1 slice whole grain bread; 1/2 cup cooked rice, pasta, or cereal; 8 crackers, 1 tortilla, muffin, or dinner roll; 1/2 bagel or hamburger bun
Milk, Cheese, Yogurt	2	3	1 cup low-fat or non-fat milk or yogurt; 1-1/2 oz cheese
Meat, Fish, Poultry, Beans, Eggs, and Nuts	2–3	4–5	1 oz cooked, lean meat, fish or chicken. Substitute 1 egg; 1/4 cup cooked peas or beans; or 1 Tbsp peanut butter for 1/2 oz of meat
Fats, Oils, and Sweets	Although dependent on size and age, fat recommendations are 60-93 gm/day or 30% of calories.		

SECTION 2
Food Sources of Selected Nutrients

Dietary Sources of Nutrients

Many patients will ask questions as to the best food sources for specific nutrients. Below and on the following pages are tables indicating dietary sources of several key nutrients.

Table 2.1 DIETARY SOURCES OF CALCIUM	
Good: >200 mg	
Food Item	Svg Size
Canned salmon w/bones	3 oz
Canned sardines w/bones	3 oz
Cheese (cheddar, edam, Monterey jack, mozzarella, Parmesan, provolone, ricotta, Romano, Swiss)	2 oz
Ice cream	1 cup
Ice milk	1 cup
Milk (skim, 2%, whole, buttermilk)	1 cup
Yogurt	1 cup
Fair 100–200 mg	
Food Item	Svg Size
Almonds	2 oz
Corn muffin	1
Cottage cheese	1 cup
Greens, collard, mustard	1/2 cup
Orange juice (calcium-fortified)	6 fl oz
Other cheeses	1 oz
Sardines	1–2 fish
Spinach	1/2 cup
Tortilla (lime-processed corn or flour)	1 (10-in. diameter)
Broccoli/Greens	1 cup

Table 2.2
DIETARY SOURCES OF FIBER*

Food Item	Svg Size	gm/Svg
Breads/Cereals/Grains		
All Bran®	1/3 cup	8.8
Bran Buds®	1/3 cup	7.9
Bran cereal	1/2 cup	8.0–13.0
Bran Chex®	2/3 cup	4.6
Cracklin' Bran®	1/2 cup	4.3
Fiber One®	1/3 cup	11.0
Oat bran	1/3 cup	4.0
Raisin bran	3/4 cup	4.0–4.8
Fruits		
Apple	1 medium	3.5
Pear	1 medium	4.1
Raspberries	1/2 cup	2.9
Strawberries	1 cup	3.0
Vegetables		
Avocado	1 medium	4.6
Baked beans	1/2 cup	8.8
Black beans	1/2 cup	5.0
Broccoli	1/2 cup	1.0
Carrots	1 cup	3.1
Green peas	1/2 cup	7.3
Kidney beans	1/2 cup	4.5
Lima beans (cooked)	1/2 cup	2.1
Pinto beans	1/2 cup	3.6
Spinach	1/2 cup	2.1
Zucchini	1/2 cup	1.8
Other		
Popcorn	3 cups	3.0
Whole wheat pasta	1 cup	3.9

*No recommended intake level has been established for children.

Table 2.3
DIETARY SOURCES OF IRON

Excellent: >4 mg

Food Item	Svg Size
Beef liver	3 oz
Clams	1/2 cup
Figs (dried)	10
Iron-fortified infant cereal	3 Tbsp.
Kidney beans	1 cup
Molasses (blackstrap)	3 Tbsp
Peaches (dried)	10 halves
Pinto beans	1 cup
Ready-to-eat, fortified cereals (like Product 19®, Total®)	3/4 cup
Sunflower seeds (dried, hulled)	2/3 cup

Good: 2–4 mg

Food Item	Svg Size
Beef	3 oz
Egg yolks	3
Iron-fortified formula	4 oz
Lamb	3 oz
Lima beans	1/2 cup
Oysters	3 oz
Peas	1 cup
Pork	3 oz
Prune juice	1 cup
Raisins	2/3 cup
Soybeans	1/2 cup

Table 2.4
DIETARY SOURCES OF POTASSIUM

Food Item	Svg Size	mg/Svg
Breads/Grains/Cereals		
Bran/All Bran®	1/3 cup	320
Fish		
Halibut	3 oz	490
Snapper	3 oz	444
Trout	3 oz	393
Fruits		
Apricot (dried)	10	482
Avocado	1	1097
Banana	1	415
Cantaloupe	1 cup	494
Carrot juice	6 oz	538
Figs (dried)	10	1332
Honeydew	1 cup	461
Mango	1 medium	322
Orange juice	8 oz	470
Papaya	1 medium	780
Prune juice	8 oz	706
Raisins	6 oz	750
Milk/Dairy		
Yogurt	6 oz	350
Vegetables		
Acorn squash	1/2 cup	446
Kidney beans	1 cup	713
Lima beans	1 cup	729
Pinto beans	1 cup	800
Potato (baked)	1 medium	844
Potato (french fried)	10 medium	366
Spinach (canned)	1/2 cup	370
Tomato juice	6 oz	400
Tomato paste	1/4 cup	550
White beans	1 cup	828
Yam	1/2 cup	455
Other		
Molasses (blackstrap)	1 Tbsp	498

Table 2.5
DIETARY SOURCES OF SODIUM

Food Item	Svg Size	mg/Svg
Breads/Grains/Cereals		
Crackers, chips (salted)	10	250
Meats		
Anchovies, sardines	3 oz	325
Bacon	3 slices	303
Ham	3.5 oz	1300
Hot dogs	1 frank	585
Bologna, other luncheon meats	1 oz slice	226
Sausage	1 link	168
Smoked meats, fish	3 oz	649
Milk/Dairy		
Buttermilk	8 oz	257
Cheese	1 oz	200–400
Cottage cheese	4 oz	457
Vegetables		
Olives	10 medium	350
Pickles, pickle relish (kosher dill)	1 oz	323
Sauerkraut	1/2 cup	780
Other		
Garlic salt	1 tsp	1300
Nuts (salted)	4 oz	700
Saladitos (salted prunes)	5	300
Salt	1 tsp	2300
Soups, bouillon (canned or dried)	8 oz	897
Soy sauce	1 oz	768

Table 2.6
DIETARY SOURCES OF VITAMIN A
(per 1/2 cup serving)

Excellent: > 3000 IU

Apricots (dried)	Papaya
Beef liver	Pumpkin
Cantaloupe	Spinach/Other dark green leafy vegetables
Carrots	
Mangoes	Squash
Mixed vegetables	

Good: 1000–3000 IU

Apricot nectar	Nectarine
Asparagus	Purple plums
Broccoli	Sweet potatoes
Chili peppers	

Fair: 500–1000 IU

Apricots (fresh)	Prunes/Prune juice
Brussels sprouts	Tomatoes/Tomato juice
Cheddar cheese	Watermelon
Peaches/Peach nectar	

Table 2.7
DIETARY SOURCES OF VITAMIN C
(per 1/2 cup serving)

Excellent: 60 mg

Broccoli	Mangoes
Brussels sprouts	Oranges/Orange juice
Cabbage	Papaya
Cauliflower	Peppers
Cranberry juice cocktail	Spinach
Grapefruit/Grapefruit juice	Strawberries
Kiwi	Vitamin C-fortified juices

Good: 25–40 mg

Asparagus	Pineapple/Pineapple juice
Bean sprouts (raw)	Potato (with skin)
Cantaloupe	Pureed baby fruits
Green chili	Tangerine
Honeydew melon	Tomatoes/Tomato juice

Table 2.8
DIETARY SOURCES OF VITAMIN D*
(per 3 oz serving)

Excellent: >100 IU (2.5 μg)

Fortified cereal	Salmon
Herring, kippers	Sardines
Mackerel	Tuna
Milk	Cod liver oil

Good: 80–100 IU (2.5 μg)

Milkshake (fast-food, Dairy Queen)	Cheese Shrimp

*Exposure to sunlight also provides vitamin D. Dark pigmented infants who are exclusively breastfed may become vitamin D deficient, particularly during winter months.

Table 2.9
DIETARY SOURCES OF VITAMIN E

Excellent: >100 IU

Food Item	Svg Size
Almonds	1 oz
Filberts	1 oz
Ready-to-eat, fortified cereals	3/4 cup
Safflower oil	1 oz
Sunflower seeds, sunflower seed oil	1 oz
Wheat germ	1 Tbsp

Good: 70–100 IU

Food Item	Svg Size
Margarine	1 oz
Olive oil	1 oz
Peanut oil	1 oz
Shrimp	1 oz
Wheat germ	1 oz

Energy and Protein Content of Selected Foods

Table 2.10 shows a listing of the energy and protein content in several commonly known types of baby foods.

Table 2.10 ENERGY AND PROTEIN CONTENT OF SELECTED BABY FOODS			
Food Items	Svg Size*	Average Calories	Average Protein (gm)
Breastmilk	1 oz	20	0.2
Formulas	1 oz	20	0.4
Cereal, infant	4 Tbsp, dry	36	1.2
Cereal, with bananas and applesauce	6 oz	183	2.6
Cereal, with bananas and apple juice	4 Tbsp, dry	60	1.0
Fruit juices	small jar (4 oz)	60	0.0
Fruit, 1st foods	2.5 oz	30–70	0.0
Fruit, 2nd foods	4.0 oz	60–90	0.6
Fruit, 3rd foods	6.0 oz	90–60	
Vegetable, 1st foods	2.5 oz	25–50	1.5
Vegetable, 2nd foods	4.0 oz	90	2.5
Meat, 2nd foods	2.5 oz	70–90	13.5
Meat, 3rd foods	2.5 oz	70–90	15.0
Meat, graduates	2.5 oz	100	8.0
Meat dinner, 2nd foods	4.0 oz	50–90	7.5
Meat dinner, 3rd foods	6.0 oz	90–130	8.0
Dessert, 2nd foods	4.0 oz	120	1.0
Dessert, 3rd foods	6.0 oz	90–150	2.5
Teething biscuit	1 biscuit	43	1.0

*2.5 oz = small jar of baby food; 4.0 oz = medium jar of baby food; 6.0 oz = large jar of baby food.

Table 2.11 shows a listing of the energy and protein content of several common food items.

Table 2.11
ENERGY AND PROTEIN CONTENT OF SELECTED COMMON FOODS

Food Group and Food Item	Svg Size	Average Calories	Average Protein (gm)
Breads and Cereals			
Bread	1 slice	80	2
Buns, biscuits, muffins	1 piece	100–200	2
Cooked cereals and grain	1/2 cup	80	2
Breakfast cereal	1 oz	90	2
Bagel	1 small	200	6
Dairy Products			
Milk, whole	8 oz	165	8
Milk, 2%	8 oz	125	8
Milk, 1%	8 oz	100	8
Milk, skim	8 oz	80	8
Cheese (cheddar, Swiss)	1 oz	120	7
Cottage cheese (2%)	1/4 cup	45	7
Yogurt, fruit flavored	8 oz	225	9
Fats			
Butter/Margarine	1 tsp	35	0
Mayonnaise	1 Tbsp	100	0
Heavy cream	1 Tbsp	52	0
Sour cream	1 Tbsp	26	0
Fruits and Vegetables			
Vegetables	1/2 cup	25	0.5–1
Fruits and fruit juices	1/2 cup	60	0.5
Protein			
Meat (fish, poultry, pork)	1 oz	35–100	7
Eggs	1	80	7
Beans (cooked)	1/2 cup	110	8
Peanut butter	2 Tbsp	190	8
Peas (cooked, split)	1/2 cup	110	8
Nuts	1 oz	170	6

Table 2.12 compares the energy density in infant foods.

Table 2.12
ENERGY CONCENTRATIONS OF STANDARD INFANT FOODS

Category	Energy Concentrations (kcals per 3-oz Serving)
Infant cereal, made with water	50
Infant cereal, made with juice	85
Infant cereal, made with breastmilk or formula	110
Infant dessert	60–95
Baby cereal in jar	55–70
Breastmilk/Formula	60
Fruit juice	40–80
Meat	90–135
Dinner high in meat	75–105
Vegetable (plain, buttered, or creamed)	25–70

Adapted from Ellyn Satter, Child of Mine: Feeding with Love and Good Sense, Bull Publishing: Palo Alto, CA, 1991.

SECTION 3
Determination of Nutrient Requirements

Recommendations for Fluid, Energy, and Protein

Calculations of fluid, energy, and protein requirements are based on the weight and age of the child (see Tables 3.1, 3.2, and 3.3).

Table 3.1 CALCULATING FLUID REQUIREMENTS	
Weight (kg*)	Fluid Requirements (cc/day)
0–10	1000
10–20	1000 + 50 cc/kg (kg >10)
>20	1500 + 20 cc/kg (kg >20)
Example: 11-month-old female	• Weight = 11 kg • Fluid = 1000cc + 50cc/kg x 1 kg • Fluid = 1050cc

Adapted from National Research Council, Recommended Dietary Allowances, 10th ed., National Academy Press: Washington, DC, 1990.

*Current weight in kilograms.

Table 3.2
CALCULATING ENERGY REQUIREMENTS

Age	Energy Requirements (kcal = kcal/kg*)
0–6 months	110
6–12 months	100
1–3 years	100
4–6 years	90
7–10 years	70
11–14 years (females)	47
11–14 years (males)	55
15–18 years (females)	40
15–18 years (males)	45
Example: 5-month-old female	• Weight = 6.5 kg • kcal/kg = 110 • kcal/day = 110 kcal/kg × 6.5 kg • kcal/day = 715

Adapted from National Research Council, Recommended Dietary Allowances, *10th ed., National Academy Press: Washington, DC, 1990.*

*Current weight in kilograms.

Table 3.3
CALCULATING PROTEIN REQUIREMENTS

Age	Protein Requirements (gm/kg*)
0–6 months	2.2
6–12 months	1.6
1–3 years	1.2
4–6 years	1.1
7–10 years	1.0
11–14 years (females)	1.0
11–14 years (males)	1.0
15–18 years (females)	0.8
15–18 years (males)	0.9

Example:	
5-month-old female	• Weight = 6.5 kg
	• Protein/kg = 2.2
	• Protein/day = 2.2 gm/kg x 6.5 kg
	• 14.3 gm

Adapted from National Research Council, Recommended Dietary Allowances, 10th ed., National Academy Press: Washington, DC, 1990.

*Current weight in kilograms.

Table 3.4
QUANTITY OF FORMULA REQUIRED TO MEET ENERGY NEEDS

Age	Weight (kg)	Formula - 20 kcal/oz
0–6 months	2	11 oz
	3	16 oz
	4	22 oz
	5	27 oz
	6	32 oz
6–12 months	7	34 oz
	8	39 oz
	9	44 oz
	10	49 oz
	11	54 oz

Most infants start eating solid foods around 4–6 months and the formula required to meet caloric needs would be reduced. This chart is a guideline in situations where a child who is older than 6 months is not eating solid foods.

SECTION 4
Assessment of Nutritional Status

Factors Associated with Nutritional Risk in Children

Children can be placed at an increased nutritional risk because of inorganic, organic, or a combination of factors.

Inorganic factors include:
- Low-income teenage mother with inadequate support system
- Mother with mental illness
- Mother with previous children with inorganic failure to thrive
- Mother with limited IQ and inadequate support system
- Economically disadvantaged family
- Child and caretaker with abnormal feeding relationship
- Child being fed a low-fat diet

Organic factors associated with diseases, inborn errors of metabolism, or birth defects may include:
- Therapeutic diets, specifically:
  –renal diets
  –low fat, low cholesterol
  –diabetic diets
- Cancer
- Cleft lip or cleft palate
- Cystic fibrosis
- Hypermetabolic states, i.e., frequent infections, burns, and heart defects

Nutritional Status Assessment

Nutritional Status Assessment (NSA) is the foundation for the provision of optimal nutritional care to pediatric patients. A complete NSA should include four *essential* components: (1) **Diet History and Evaluation**, (2) **Anthropometric Measurements**, (3) **Biochemical Evaluation**, and (4) **Nutrition Physical Examination** (see Table 4.1). These four components provide direction for the development of an effective, appropriate, and individualized nutritional care plan for the child. No single component of the NSA is adequate to make a nutritional diagnosis.

Nutritional assessment data should be re-evaluated on a regular basis to provide an in-depth understanding of the child's nutritional needs. This section of the manual provides information on evaluating the diet history, anthropometric measurements, and laboratory values obtained in an NSA. The nutrition physical examination in pediatrics primarily focuses on physical examination for signs of muscle wasting, dehydration, obesity, or pale mucous membranes associated with iron-deficiency anemia.

Figure 4.1 is a chart to organize the collection of data for nutrition status assessment.

Table 4.1
KEY COMPONENTS OF THE NUTRITIONAL STATUS ASSESSMENT

Diet History and Evaluation
- 24-hour recall
- Food allergies, preferences, intolerances
- Food frequency
- Related medical history
- Usual eating pattern
- Weight history

Anthropometric Measurements
- Weight
- Height/Length
- Head circumference
- Mid-arm muscle circumference
- Triceps skinfolds

Biochemical Evaluation
- Electrolytes
- Indicators of fluid status
- Indicators of mineral status (i.e., iron, etc.)
- Vitamin/Micronutrient levels
- Indicators of substrate (carbohydrate, protein, or fat) intolerance
- Visceral protein stores

Nutrition Physical Examination
- Hair
- Skin
- Nails
- Eyes
- Oral (tongue and gums)
- Lips/Mucous membranes
- Overall musculature, adipose stores

Figure 4.1
NUTRITION STATUS ASSESSMENT FORM

Name: _____ Date: _____ Room #: _____
Patient Number: _____ Age: _____ Sex: _____
Physician: _____ Diet Rx: _____

ANTHROPOMETRIC

Height/Length: _____ %tile: _____
Weight: _____ %tile: _____
UBW: _____
TSF: ___ %tile: ___ MAC: ___ %tile: ___
MAMC: _____ %tile: _____
Other: _____
HC: _____ %tile: _____
Weight-for-Height %tile: _____

BIOCHEMICAL EVALUATION

Albumin: _____
Hemoglobin: _____
Hematocrit: _____
HDL Cholesterol: _____
LDL Cholesterol: _____
Other: _____

DIET HISTORY

Breakfast: _____

Lunch: _____

Dinner: _____

Snacks: _____

Breastfeeding/Formula Regime: _____

NUTRITION PHYSICAL

General:

Oral/Mucosa:

Other Signs:

SUMMARY AND RECOMMENDATIONS:

Adapted with permission from Arizona Dietetic Association, Inc., Arizona Diet Manual, Arizona Dietetic Association: Phoenix, AZ, 1992.

Evaluating Growth

The single most sensitive and specific indicator of malnutrition in children is their growth. Height/Length and weight are the most sensitive anthropometric measurements in the pediatric population. As infancy and childhood are periods of very rapid growth, malnutrition will quickly affect growth rate and potential. Growth is most optimally evaluated over a period of time, by using the NCHS growth charts (Figures 4.2 to 4.9) for height/length, weight, and head circumference.

Growth assessments should be completed during all medical evaluations. Until the age of 2 years, a child's height/length is measured while the child is lying on a board (use growth charts for birth to 36 months of age). After 2 years of age, height is measured while the child is standing on a stadiometer (use growth charts for 2 to 18 years of age). From birth to 18 months of age, a child's weight is measured without clothes or diapers; after 18 months of age, with clothes but no shoes).

The NCHS growth charts have been developed by observing large populations over time. The percentile line closest to the child's measurements provides a value indicating how the child's growth compares with the population as a whole. Small children follow the lower percentiles, and large children the upper percentiles. Normal growth rates follow along the same percentile lines over time. Deviation from normal growth occurs when a child's growth rate increases or decreases by more than two major percentiles, either higher or lower (i.e., from the 25th percentile to the 75th percentile). Statistically, 10% of children will plot below or above the curve lines. Monitoring these indicators longitudinally is an acceptable method for evaluating growth status. Some variation in growth is seen between breastfed versus formula-fed infants (see Weight Gain Velocity for Breastfed Infants , Section 6).

Average Weight Gain

Table 4.2 is helpful for evaluating weight gain on an individual basis. This is the *mean* growth rate; rates will vary for smaller or larger children. This table is most useful for children who do not follow the growth curve or who need to be evaluated on a daily basis.

Table 4.2
AVERAGE WEIGHT GAIN

Age (mos, years)	Grams/Day	Grams/Month	Kilograms/Year
0–3	30	1000	—
4–6	20	850	—
7–9	15	500	—
10–12	12	360	—
13–18	7	200	—
19–24	6	180	—
25–30	6	180	—
31–35	6	180	—
3–10 years	7	200	2.5
11–14 years (females)	12.5	375	4.5
11–15 years (males)	15	460	5.5

Growth Charts

Figures 4.2 through 4.9 were developed by the National Center for Health Statistics in collaboration with the Centers for Disease Control. They are based on data from national probability samples representative of children in the general population. They are useful to record the growth of individual children and identify unusual growth patterns which may be due to poor nutrition or illness.

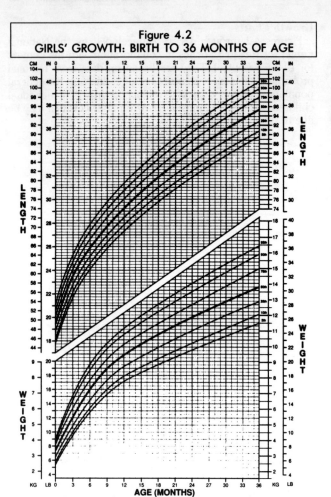

Figure 4.2 GIRLS' GROWTH: BIRTH TO 36 MONTHS OF AGE

*Adapted from: Hamill PVV, Drizd TA, Johnson CL, Reed RB, Roche AF, Moore WM: Physical growth: National Center for Health Statistics percentiles. AM J CLIN NUTR 32:607–629, 1979. Data from the National Center for Health Statistics (NCHS), Hyattsville, Maryland. © 1982 Ross Laboratories

Assessment of Nutritional Status

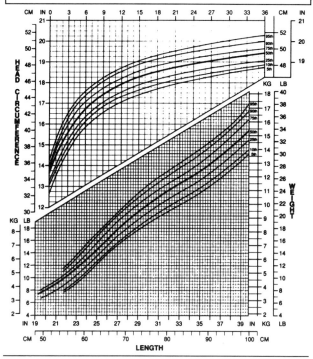

**Figure 4.3
GIRLS' WEIGHT FOR LENGTH: BIRTH TO 36 MONTHS OF AGE**

*Adapted from: Hamill PVV, Drizd TA, Johnson CL, Reed RB, Roche AF, Moore WM: Physical growth: National Center for Health Statistics percentiles. AM J CLIN NUTR 32:607–629, 1979. Data from the National Center for Health Statistics (NCHS), Hyattsville, Maryland. © 1982 Ross Laboratories

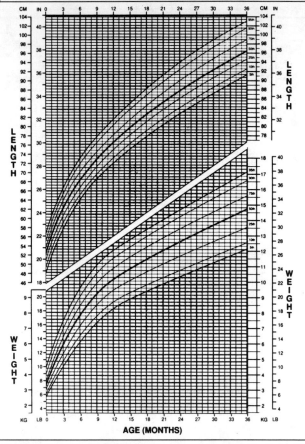

Figure 4.4
BOYS' GROWTH: BIRTH TO 36 MONTHS OF AGE

*Adapted from: Hamill PVV, Drizd TA, Johnson CL, Reed RB, Roche AF, Moore WM: Physical growth: National Center for Health Statistics percentiles. AM J CLIN NUTR 32:607–629, 1979. Data from the National Center for Health Statistics (NCHS), Hyattsville, Maryland. © 1982 Ross Laboratories

Assessment of Nutritional Status 45

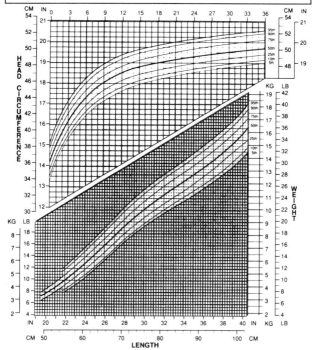

Figure 4.5
BOYS' WEIGHT FOR LENGTH: BIRTH TO 36 MONTHS OF AGE

*Adapted from: Hamill PVV, Drizd TA, Johnson CL, Reed RB, Roche AF, Moore WM: Physical growth: National Center for Health Statistics percentiles. AM J CLIN NUTR 32:607–629, 1979. Data from the National Center for Health Statistics (NCHS), Hyattsville, Maryland. © 1982 Ross Laboratories

46 Pediatric Nutrition Handbook

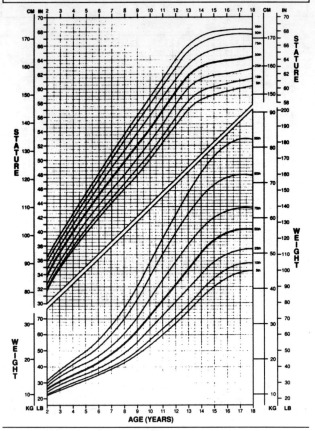

*Adapted from: Hamill PVV, Drizd TA, Johnson CL, Reed RB, Roche AF, Moore WM: Physical growth: National Center for Health Statistics percentiles. AM J CLIN NUTR 32:607–629, 1979. Data from the National Center for Health Statistics (NCHS), Hyattsville, Maryland. © 1982 Ross Laboratories

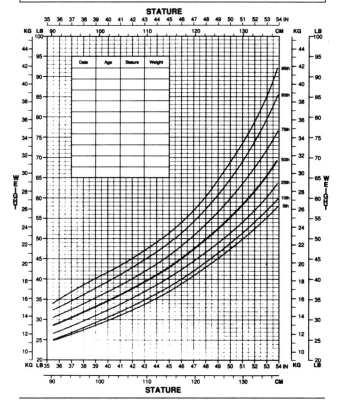

Figure 4.7
GIRLS' WEIGHT FOR HEIGHT: 2 TO 12 YEARS OF AGE

*Adapted from: Hamill PVV, Drizd TA, Johnson CL, Reed RB, Roche AF, Moore WM: Physical growth: National Center for Health Statistics percentiles. AM J CLIN NUTR 32:607–629, 1979. Data from the National Center for Health Statistics (NCHS), Hyattsville, Maryland. © 1982 Ross Laboratories

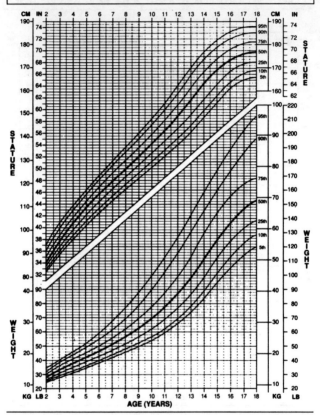

**Figure 4.8
BOYS' GROWTH: 2 TO 18 YEARS OF AGE**

*Adapted from: Hamill PVV, Drizd TA, Johnson CL, Reed RB, Roche AF, Moore WM: Physical growth: National Center for Health Statistics percentiles. AM J CLIN NUTR 32:607–629, 1979. Data from the National Center for Health Statistics (NCHS), Hyattsville, Maryland. © 1982 Ross Laboratories

Figure 4.9
BOYS' WEIGHT FOR HEIGHT: 2 TO 12 YEARS OF AGE

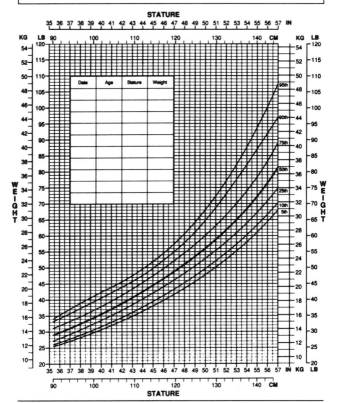

*Adapted from: Hamill PVV, Drizd TA, Johnson CL, Reed RB, Roche AF, Moore WM: Physical growth: National Center for Health Statistics percentiles. AM J CLIN NUTR 32:607–629, 1979. Data from the National Center for Health Statistics (NCHS), Hyattsville, Maryland. © 1982 Ross Laboratories

Other Methods for Measuring Growth

Skinfold thickness is an indicator of body fat content. Approximately one-half of the body's adipose tissue is located in subcutaneous areas. The most reproducible sites that are measured include the triceps, subscapular, abdominal, hip, and thigh skinfolds. These measurements are taken with calipers and are more accurate when completed by someone who is well trained and experienced in anthropometric techniques. Triceps measurements are often used to evaluate fat mass and longitudinal fat mass changes. Figure 4.10 demonstrates the measurement of the triceps skinfolds. Table 4.3 provides percentiles for triceps skinfolds for Caucasians in the United States.

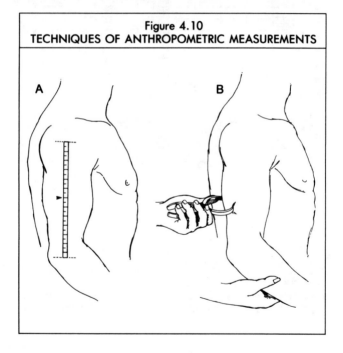

Figure 4.10
TECHNIQUES OF ANTHROPOMETRIC MEASUREMENTS

Table 4.3
PERCENTILES FOR TRICEPS SKINFOLDS FOR WHITES OF THE U.S.

Age (yr)	Triceps Skinfold Percentiles (mm^2) — Males						
	5	10	25	50	75	90	95
1–1.9	6	7	8	10	12	14	16
2–2.9	6	7	8	10	12	14	15
3–3.9	6	7	8	10	11	14	15
4–4.9	6	6	8	9	11	12	14
5–5.9	6	6	8	9	11	14	15
6–6.9	5	6	7	8	10	13	16
7–7.9	5	6	7	9	12	15	17
8–8.9	5	6	7	8	10	13	16
9–9.9	6	6	7	10	13	17	18
10–10.9	6	6	8	10	14	18	21
11–11.9	6	6	8	11	16	20	24
12–12.9	6	6	8	11	14	22	28
13–13.9	5	5	7	10	14	22	26
14–14.9	4	5	7	9	14	21	24
15–15.9	4	5	6	8	11	18	24
16–16.9	4	5	6	8	12	16	22
17–17.9	5	5	6	8	12	16	19
18–18.9	4	5	6	9	13	20	24

Health and Nutrition Examination Survey I of 1971 to 1974. Adapted from Frisancho, A.R. New Norms of Upper Limb Fat and Muscle Areas for Assessment of Nutritional Status. Am J Clin Nutr 34:2540, 1981.

Data collected from whites in the United States Health and Nutrition Examination Survey I (1971–1974).

continued on next page

Table 4.3
PERCENTILES FOR TRICEPS SKINFOLDS FOR WHITES OF THE U.S. *Continued*

Triceps Skinfold Percentiles (mm^2)

Age (yr)	Females						
	5	10	25	50	75	90	95
1–1.9	6	7	8	10	12	14	16
2–2.9	6	8	9	10	12	15	16
3–3.9	7	8	9	11	12	14	15
4–4.9	7	8	8	10	12	14	16
5–5.9	6	7	8	10	12	15	18
6–6.9	6	6	8	10	12	14	16
7–7.9	6	7	9	11	13	16	18
8–8.9	6	8	9	12	15	18	24
9–9.9	8	8	10	13	16	20	22
10–10.9	7	8	10	12	17	23	27
11–11.9	7	8	10	13	18	24	28
12–12.9	8	9	11	14	18	23	27
13–13.9	8	8	12	15	21	26	30
14–14.9	9	10	13	16	21	26	28
15–15.9	8	10	12	17	21	25	32
16–16.9	10	12	15	18	22	26	31
17–17.9	10	12	13	19	24	30	37
18–18.9	10	12	15	18	22	26	30

Health and Nutrition Examination Survey I of 1971 to 1974. Adapted from Frisancho, A.R. New Norms of Upper Limb Fat and Muscle Areas for Assessment of Nutritional Status. Am J Clin Nutr 34:2540, 1981.

Data collected from whites in the United States Health and Nutrition Examination Survey I (1971–1974).

Assessment of Inadequate Growth: "Failure to Thrive"

Definition of Failure to Thrive
- Weight-for-height ratio below the 5th percentile on the NCHS growth curve charts.
- Actual weight 20% or more below the ideal weight-for-height.
- Poor weight gain:
  −20 gm/day or less from birth to 3 months
  −15 gm/day or less from 3 to 6 months
- Crossing two major percentiles on the NCHS growth curve charts; for example, dropping from the 75th percentile to the 25th percentile

Causes of Failure to Thrive
Infants and children may experience inadequate growth (failure to thrive) from such causes as malabsorption, cystic fibrosis, tropical sprue, restrictive diets for allergies, inborn errors of metabolism, inadequate provision of food, and frequent illnesses (see also Factors Associated with Nutritional Risk in Children, Section 4, pg 35).

Severity Classifications of Failure to Thrive
(Tables 4.4 and 4.5)

Table 4.4
CALCULATING PERCENT OF STANDARD WEIGHT FOR HEIGHT

% of standard* =	Actual Weight % by weight-for-height at the 50th percentile
	Example: 12-month-old male • length: 77.0 cm • weight: 8.7 kg • weight-for-height at 50th percentile = 10.3 kg
% of standard* =	$\dfrac{8.7 \text{ kg}}{10.3 \text{ kg}} = 84\%$ (mild)

*Compare % of standard on Waterlow Classification Chart (Table 4.5).

Table 4.5
WATERLOW CLASSIFICATION CHART

Grade of Malnutrition	Weight-for-Height (% of Standard)
0	> 90
1 = mild	80–89
2 = moderate	70–80
3 = severe	< 70

Waterlow Classification Chart. British Medical Journal 3:112, 566–569, 1972.

Assessment of Excessive Fat Stores: "Obesity"

Definition of Obesity
Obesity is excess body fat (weight-for-height above the 95th percentile). Unfortunately, no ideal technique for diagnosing obesity currently exists.

Assessment of Obesity
Table 4.6 reveals some of the current methods for evaluating obesity. **NOTE:** The ***distribution of fat*** is more important than the ***total fat*** in determining risk for obesity-related disorders in children.

Estimation of Normal Height and Weight
The following equations are estimations to use when height and weight measurement tools are unavailable:

Height (inches)
Age 2–14 years—(age in yrs x 2.5) + 30

Weight (pounds)
Age 1–6 years—(age in yrs x 5) + 17
Age 6–12 years—(age in yrs x 7) + 5

Laboratory Assessment of Nutritional Status

Laboratory evaluation is occasionally used in pediatric medicine and usually focuses on the periodic evaluation of anemia. Tables 4.7 through 4.12 (on pgs 56 to 64) provide relevant data to effectively and accurately evaluate laboratory data for a pediatric patient population.

Table 4.6
BODY FAT ASSESSMENT METHODS

Method	Positive Aspects	Negative Aspects
Weight	• Convenient, reproducible standards are available.	• Not independent of height. • Does not assess fat distribution. • Poorly correlated with morbidity.
Body Mass Index (BMI) ($wt \div ht^2$)	• Convenient, reproducible standards are available. • Independent of height.	• Does not assess fat distribution. • Poorly correlated with morbidity.
Skinfolds	• Standards are available. • Independent of height. • Assesses fat distribution. • Correlated with morbidity.	• Reproducible only with trained measurers. • Requires calipers.
Densitometry (underwater weighing)	• Considered "gold standard." • Standards are available. • Correlated with morbidity.	• Not convenient. • Does not assess fat distribution. • Requires extensive equipment.

Table 4.7
EVALUATION OF ANEMIA

Test	Specimen	Reference	Mean Normal Range*
Ferritin**	Serum		ng/ml
		Newborn:	25–200
		1 month:	200–600
		2–5 months:	50–200
		6 months–15 years:	7–140
Hematocrit** (Hct)	Whole Blood (EDTA)		% of packed red cells
		1 day (cap):	48–69
		2 days:	48–75
		3 days:	44–72
		2 months:	28–42
		6–12 years:	35–45
			Males / Females
		12–18 years:	37–49 / 36–46

*Mean normal range will vary with laboratory used. Check your laboratory for specific information.

**Calculated from MCV & RBC. Percent of packed red cells (volume red cells/volume whole blood × 100).

Source: Textbook of Pediatrics, W.B. Saunders, Philadelphia, 1992.

Table 4.7 EVALUATION OF ANEMIA Continued

Test	Specimen	Reference	Mean Normal Range*
Hemoglobin (Hgb)	Whole Blood (EDTA)		*g/dL*
		1–3 day (cap):	14.5–22.5
		2 months:	9.0–14.0
		6–12 years:	11.5–15.5
			Males *Females*
		12–18 years:	13.0–16.0 12.0–16.0
Iron	Serum		*µg/dL*
		Newborn:	100–250
		Infant:	40–100
		Child:	50–120
			Males *Females*
		Thereafter:	50–160 40–150
		Intoxicated child:	280–2550
		Fatally poisoned child:	>1800
Mean Corpuscular Hemoglobin Concentration (MCHC)	Whole Blood (EDTA)		*% Hgb/cell or gm Hgb/dL RBC*
		Birth:	30–60
		1–3 (cap):	29–37
		1–2 weeks:	28–38
		1–2 months:	29–37
		3 months–2 years:	30–36
		2–18 years:	31–37

Table 4.7 EVALUATION OF ANEMIA *Continued*

Test	Specimen	Reference	Mean Normal Range*
Mean Corpuscular Volume (MCV)	Whole Blood	1–3 day (cap): 0.5–2 years: 6–12 years: 12–18 years:	μm^3 95–121 70–86 77–95 Males Females 78–98 78–102
Total Iron Binding Capacity (TIBC)	Serum	Infant: Thereafter	$\mu g/dl$ 100–400 250–400
Transferrin	Serum	Newborn: Thereafter:	mg/dl 218–347 208–378
Vitamin B_{12}	Serum	Newborn: Thereafter:	pg/dl 175–800 140–700

*Mean normal range will vary with laboratory used. Check your laboratory for specific information.

Source: *Textbook of Pediatrics*, W.B. Saunders, Philadelphia, 1992.

Table 4.8
CALCIUM ABNORMALITIES

Test	Specimen	Reference		Mean Range
Ionized Calcium	Serum, Plasma, or Whole Blood (Heparin)	*Fasting*		*mg/dL*
			Cord:	5.0–6.0
			Newborn, 3–24 hours:	4.3–5.1
			Newborn, 24–48 hours:	4.0–4.7
			Thereafter:	4.48–4.92
Total Calcium	Serum	*Age*		*mg/dL*
			Cord:	9.0–11.5
			Newborn, 3–24 hours:	9.0–10.6
			Newborn, 24–48 hours:	7.0–12.0
			Newborn, 4–7 days:	9.0–10.9
			Child:	8.8–10.8
			Thereafter:	8.4–10.2
	Urine, 24-hour	*Calcium in diet*		*mg/dL*
			Diet calcium-free:	5–40
			Low to average:	50–150
			Average:	100–300

Table 4.9
CARBOHYDRATE ABNORMALITIES

Test	Specimen	Reference	Mean Normal Range	
Glucose	Serum	Fasting	mg/dL	
		Cord:	45–96	
		Premature:	20–60	
		Neonate:	30–60	
		Newborn, 1 day:	40–60	
		Newborn, >1 day:	50–90	
		Child:	60–100	
Glucose Tolerance Test**	Serum		mg/dL	
			Normal	Diabetic
		Fasting:	70–105	>115
		60 min.:	120–170	≥200
		90 min.:	100–140	≥200
		120 min.:	70–120	≥140
H_2 Breath Test*** for Lactose Malabsorption	Exhaled Breath	Abnormal:	H_2 excretion >20 ppm above baseline	

*Mean normal range will vary with laboratory used. Check your laboratory for specific information.

**Oral glucose dose in the Glucose Tolerance Test for children is 1.75 gm/kg ideal weight up to a maximum of 75 gm.

***H_2 breath t-test dose: 2 gm/kg of 20% lactose solution up to 50 gm.

Table 4.10
LIPID ASSESSMENT

Test	Specimen	Reference	Mean Normal Range*	
			mg/dL	
Fat Malabsorption Triglycerides	Serum, after ≥ 12-hour fast		Males	Females
		Cord blood:	10–98	10–98
		0-5 years:	30–86	32–99
		6–11 years:	31–108	35–14
		12–15 years:	36–138	41–38
		16–19 years:	40–163	40–128
			Coefficient of fat absorption (%)	
Fecal Fat	Feces, 72-hour	Infant, breastfed:	>93	
		Infant, formula-fed:	>83	
		>1 year:	≥95	
			mg/dL	
HDL Cholesterol	Serum or Plasma (EDTA)		Males	Females
		Cord blood:	5–50	5–50
		0–12 years:	30–65	30–65
		15–19 years:	30–65	30–70
			mg/dL	
LDL Cholesterol	Serum or Plasma (EDTA)		Males	Females
		Cord blood:	10–50	10–50
		0–19 years:	60–140	60–150

*Mean normal range with laboratory used. Check with your laboratory for specific information.

Table 4.11
PROTEIN MALNUTRITION

Test	Specimen	Reference	Mean Normal Range*
Albumin	Serum		*g/dL*
		Premature:	1.8–3.0
		Newborn:	2.5–3.4
		Infant:	4.0–5.0
		Thereafter:	3.5–5.0
Prealbumin (Thyroxine-binding)	Serum		*mg/dL*
		Cord:	13
		1 years:	12–27
		2–18 years:	10–40
Total Protein	Serum		*g/dL*
		Premature:	4.3–7.6
		Newborn:	4.6–7.4
		Child:	6.2–8.0

*Mean normal range will vary with laboratory used. Check with your laboratory for specific information.

Table 4.12
OTHER EVALUATIONS OF NUTRITIONAL STATUS

Test	Specimen	Reference	Mean Normal Range*
Lead	Whole Blood (Heparin)	Child:	*µg/dL* <10
Potassium	Serum		*mmol/L*
		Newborn:	3.9–5.9
		Infant:	4.1–5.3
		Child:	3.4–4.7
		Thereafter:	3.5–5.1

*Mean normal range will vary with laboratory used. Check with your laboratory for specific information.

SECTION 5
Referral Criteria

Nutritional Referral

Indications for Nutrition Referral
- Failure to thrive.
- Weight-for-height below the 5th percentile on the NCHS standard growth curve charts.
- Actual weight 20% or more below the ideal weight-for-height.
- Poor weight gain:
    20 gm/day or less from birth to 3 months of age; or
    15 gm/day or less from 3 to 6 months.
- Any disease or therapy requiring a therapeutic diet.
- Inborn errors of metabolism.
- Infant that starts solids before 3 months.
- Infant with normal development who has not started solids by 8 months.
- Food allergies.
- Cystic fibrosis.
- Obesity.
- Hypercholesterolemia.
- Vegetarianism, especially if this is a new style of eating for family. Not necessary in cases of traditional vegetarian diet.
- Athlete or adolescent on restricted diet.
- Child on medication which interferes with nutrients.

Writing Nutrition Referrals/Consults

Sample Referrals

The following are sample referrals to assist in formulating patient referrals to nutrition. Referrals should be clear and concise, providing any pertinent data for assessment and specifying the outcome desired.

1. **Failure to Thrive:** 3-y/o male with inadequate growth in last year. Weight has dropped from the 75th percentile to the 10th percentile. Height remains constant at the 75th percentile. Growth chart enclosed. Evaluate diet and prescribe appropriate nutritional and behavior therapy to increase energy intake.
2. **Iron-Deficiency Anemia:** 1.5-y/o female with iron-deficiency anemia, H/H 10.0/29.0, serum Fe^+ 42, and serum ferritin 8. Patient is unable to tolerate $FeSO_4$ supplement due to severe G.I. distress. Constipation. Evaluate diet for nutritional adequacy, and educate patient's mother about increasing iron, as well as strategies to reduce G.I. distress.
3. **Obesity:** 11-y/o female. Height 5'0". Weight 120 lbs. Strong family history of obesity and related diseases. Evaluate diet and activity pattern and prescribe appropriate nutritional therapy to stabilize weight gain.

Supplemental Feeding Programs for Women, Infants, and Children

The U.S. federal government currently funds two comprehensive nutrition programs for pregnant women, infants, and children: (1) the Women, Infants, and Children (WIC) Program, and (2) Food Plus. These programs are administered at the county level and are summarized in Table 5.1.

Other Referral Agencies
1. Local health department
2. Local hospital nutrition department
3. American Dietetic Association, Consumer Nutrition Hotline and Nationwide Nutrition Network (1-800-366-1655)

Table 5.1
SUMMARY OF TWO SUPPLEMENTAL FEEDING PROGRAMS

	WIC*	Food Plus
Target Audience	• Pregnant women • Breastfeeding women • Non-breastfeeding mothers of infants <6 months old • Infants <1 year • Children <5 years	• Pregnant women • Breastfeeding women • Non-breastfeeding mothers of infants <1 year old • No infants • Children <6 years old
Purpose	• Provide nutritious foods, health checks, referrals, nutrition education, and counseling	• Provide nutrient-rich foods and nutrition education
Eligibility	• Low income: <185% federal poverty level for women and children • County resident • Health risk (anemia, poor diet, etc.)	• Low income: <185% federal poverty level for women and children • County resident • No health risk
Food	• Nutrient-rich • Limited brand names • Patient-purchased food from local supermarkets ($45/month)	• Nutrient-rich • Government-purchased brand names and commodities • Warehouse distribution of 50 lbs/month
Nutrition Education	• Individual and group • Specific to risk	• Food demonstrations • Newsletters, recipes
Health Checks	• Height, weight, and anemia testing for women, infants, and children	• Height, weight, and anemia testing for women and children

Adapted from information provided by the Pima County (Arizona) Health Department.

*WIC = Women, Infant & Children Supplemental government feeding program.

SECTION 6
Age-Specific Recommendations

Feeding Infants

Breastfeeding Basics

A women's ability to breastfeed is influenced by her confidence and support during the first weeks and months of her child's life. Health care providers should serve as a significant source of counseling and encouragement for new mothers.

Algorithm for Successful Breastfeeding

The mechanical success of breastfeeding depends on the child's ability to stimulate the breast, ingest, digest, and metabolize the milk, and the mother's ability to produce and provide adequate access to the milk. One of the most important facts to know about breastfeeding is that it works on *a law of supply and demand*. Frequent and unrestricted access to the breast will determine the amount of breastmilk produced. Intervention, such as formula supplementation or pacifiers, will interfere with the infant's desire or ability to breastfeed. This will reduce milk production. The breastfeeding algorithm (Figure 6.1) details the components of successful breastfeeding.

Advantages of Breastfeeding
- Breastmilk is nutritionally superior to any alternative.
- Breastmilk contains immunoglobulins and maternal antibodies, including macro-phages, lymphocytes, B-cells, T-cells, and secretory IgA.
- Breastmilk is bacteriologically safe, always fresh, and requires no preparation.
- Breastmilk is the least allergenic of any infant food.
- Breastfed infants have lower rates of diarrhea and other infections, including otitis media.
- Breastmilk promotes G.I. tract maturation.
- Breastfeeding promotes jaw and tooth development.
- Breastfed babies are less likely to be overfed.

- Breastfeeding may decrease a woman's risk for breast cancer.
- Breastmilk is less expensive than formula.
- Breastfeeding promotes infant-maternal bonding.
- Although postpartum weight loss occurs at a similar rate, breastfeeding women lose proportionally more body fat mass than do non-breastfeeding women.
- Breastfed infants appear to have advanced intellectual performance at age 5 years.

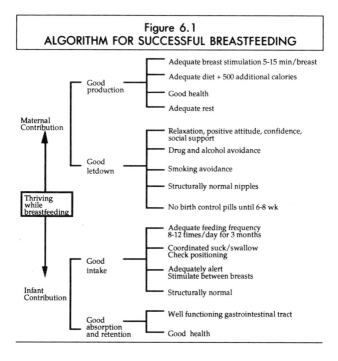

Figure 6.1
ALGORITHM FOR SUCCESSFUL BREASTFEEDING

Weight Gain Velocity for Breastfed Infants

The pattern of velocity and composition of weight gain is different between breastfed and formula-fed infants, who are the basis for the NCHS growth charts. Breastfed infants tend to gain less weight the first few weeks after birth compared with bottle-fed infants. Breastfed infants may then have a greater velocity of weight gain until about 3-4 months of age when the pattern of their weight gain equals bottle-fed infants. After 4 months of age, breastfed infants tend to gain weight more slowly compared with formula-fed infants. The difference in weights appears to be a result of less adipose tissue storage in breastfed infants without any associated risk of increased morbidity.

Health care professionals must be aware of these differences to prevent misdiagnosing normal growth as an insufficient supply of breastmilk, thus encouraging formula supplements and decreasing breast stimulation and milk production.

Breastmilk Storage

Working mothers can successfully breastfeed by using manual or electric breast pumps. Table 6.1 provides safe storage times for breastmilk.

Table 6.1 SAFE STORAGE TIMES FOR BREASTMILK		
Storage	*Freshly Expressed Breastmilk*	*Previously Frozen Breastmilk*
Freezer	• 6 months (separate door refrigerator/freezer) • 12 months or longer (deep freezer)	Do not refreeze
Refrigerator	72 hours	24 hours
Room Temperature (<80°F)	6—10 hours*	Do not store

*Although acceptable, refrigeration is preferable.

Developed by Pat Bull, Breastmilk Collection and Storage, Medela, Inc.: McHenry, IL, 1994.

Recommendations for Working Mothers[*]

The following suggestions are helpful for mothers who return to work:

- Pump in the morning when breasts are full. Breastfeed on one side, then immediately pump the other. To increase milk supply, let the baby breastfeed on the side just pumped.
- By 3–4 weeks postpartum, most lactating mothers produce about 25 oz of milk a day. Even then, some mothers may only express 2 oz at a time.
- Give the baby expressed milk in a bottle at about 3-6 weeks of age.
- Freeze expressed breastmilk in 2- to 3-oz portions. Also freeze 1/2- to 1-oz portions, in case the baby may want a little more. When the baby is older, freeze milk in 4-oz portions.
- After the milk supply is well established, use formula as a backup in emergencies. Be careful though: If formula is given on a regular basis, milk production will decrease.

How to Respond to Concerns of Lactating Women

Breastfeeding mothers may need help in addressing their concerns related to lactation and breastfeeding. Table 6.2 offers some appropriate breastfeeding tips. In addition, certain medications may be contraindicated during lactation (see Table 6.3).

Foods and Beverages Which May Cause Infant G.I. Distress

There are no foods which should be routinely avoided, but occasionally an infant will be bothered by something the mother has eaten. Many mothers will become aware of what foods bother their infant. Cultures have different attitudes and behaviors about what breastfeeding mothers should eat and how food affects infants. These changes should be discussed with mothers to inform and encourage the most balance in food selections. Reviewing the previous day's food intakes may be needed for women who mention that their infant sometimes refuses the breast. Table 6.4 contains a list of some possibly problematic foods and beverages.

If an infant has frequent colic, the mother should be advised to avoid the foods listed in Table 6.4 on a trial basis in order to determine if a change in diet reduces infant colic. If whole food groups are omitted, the mother should see a dietitian to assure adequate nutrition.

*Adapted from Nutrition and Your Child, *Baylor College of Medicine, Children's Nutrition Research Center, Spring 1993.*

Table 6.2
BREASTFEEDING TIPS

Concern	Recommended Action
Breast Care	Nipple pulling, tugging, or rolling during pregnancy is not necessary to prepare for breastfeeding. Avoid soaps or lotions to the nipples. Air dry nipples after breastfeeding.
Breast Creams	Vitamin E, breast creams, or ointments are not recommended. They have not been shown to heal the nipple and can make soreness worse by keeping the nipple moist (see "Nipples, Sore").
Breast Surgery	Any type of breast surgery may interfere with milk supply. Consult with a lactation consultant and/or your doctor for individual advice.
Cesarean Section (C-section)	Breastfeed your baby as soon as possible after delivery, preferably in the recovery room. Hold your baby in a comfortable position. Use pillows across your abdomen to protect the incision and support the baby. You will need additional rest and support at home.
Duration of Breastfeeding: How long and how often?	Breastfeed every 2–3 hours for at least 10–15 minutes on each breast. Watch your baby for signs that he is full, like falling asleep, losing interest in feeding, or stopping breastfeeding. Your breast is never completely empty. It is alright to switch breasts several times during a feeding.
Early First Feeding	Put baby to your breast soon after delivery, if possible within the first 2 hours. Cuddling, licking, and brief sucking are good signs that you and your baby are learning to breastfeed. Offer your breast often to let your baby practice. Ask a supportive nurse for help.

Table 6.2 BREASTFEEDING TIPS *Continued*

Concern	Recommended Action
Engorgement	Engorgement may occur when milk first comes in or when feedings are missed or delayed. Use warm compresses or take a hot shower before feedings. Hand express to soften areola, making it easier for baby to latch on. Breastfeed every 1–2 hours for 10–20 minutes per breast. If unable to breastfeed, pump milk to relieve pressure. Apply ice to breast and under arm after feeding until swelling decreases. Take non-aspirin pain reliever. If no relief in 48 hours, call lactation consultant or doctor.
Extra Feedings	Healthy breastfed newborns do not need formula, water, or juice. Breastfeed at least every 2-3 hours during the first month. Older breastfed babies will be ready for solid foods and juices between 4–6 months of age.
Fussy Infant	If no indication of illness, reassure, discuss growth spurts, development. Determine time of fussiness; every evening 4–8 pm normal irritable time. During growth spurts, infants who were sleeping through the night may revert to waking to nurse. This is good; stimulates production.
Hospital Survival Skills	"Rooming-in" with your baby is your right as a consumer. Keep your baby with you as much as possible so you can breastfeed often. Do not give bottles. Do not limit feeding time at your breast. Ask a supportive nurse for help. Do not accept formula gift packs.
Inadequate Supply	Frequent nursing: 10–15 minutes/breast. Check mom's diet, exercise, rest, medical history, medications, babies birth history.

continued on next page

Table 6.2
BREASTFEEDING TIPS *Continued*

Concern	Recommended Action
Is Baby Getting Enough Milk?	Your body makes as much milk as your baby needs. Signs that a newborn is getting enough breast milk are: 6–8 wet diapers a day, baby sleeps some between feedings; and baby gains 3–7 oz/week. Babies less than 4 weeks old should have at least one bowel movement a day. Older babies may go 3–4 days between bowel movements.
Jaundice	Try to breastfeed at least every 2 hours around the clock. If breastfeeding is stopped, pump your breasts to maintain milk supply. Avoid water or formula feedings. Consult your baby's doctor.
Latch-on	Latch-on is necessary for baby to begin sucking at your breast. Poor latch-on is a major cause of sore nipples. Baby's mouth should be at nipple level. Support your breast by placing the thumb on the top and four fingers underneath. Tickle baby's bottom lip with nipple until baby opens mouth very wide. Center your nipple quickly and bring the baby very close to you. Baby's nose and chin should be touching breast.
Leaking	Leaking is a sign of normal letdown in the early weeks of breastfeeding. You may use breast pads in your bra between feedings. Avoid pads with plastic lining. During sexual activity, leaking may occur; you may wish to breastfeed the baby first.

Table 6.2
BREASTFEEDING TIPS *Continued*

Concern	Recommended Action
Mastitis	Mastitis is a swollen, inflamed, or infected area in the breast. Watch for flu-like symptoms such as fever above 101°F; chills and muscle aches; and a reddened, hot, tender or swollen area in the breast. Rest, breastfeed often, and drink more fluids. Contact your doctor as antibiotics may be needed. Do not stop breastfeeding.
Mother's Concerns	Provide quantitative reassurances (i.e., weight gain, and/or 6–8 wet diapers/day is good indicator of adequate supply once milk is established).
Myths and Misconception	The truth is: Breast sagging is not a result of breastfeeding. Breast size does not affect ability to breastfeed. Drinking beer, Manzanilla tea, or large amounts of fluids does not make more milk.
Nipples, Flat or Inverted (before birth)	Flat or inverted nipples retract or move in toward the breast. Breast shells (milk cups) may be worn during pregnancy to help minimize inverted nipples. Gradually increase time of use from a few hours to 8–10 hours/day. Do not wear while sleeping. Air dry nipples if leaking occurs. Breast shells should not be used by women at risk for preterm labor. Check with your doctor.

continued on next page

Table 6.2 BREASTFEEDING TIPS *Continued*

Concern	Recommended Action
Nipples, Flat or Inverted (after birth)	Begin breastfeeding as soon as possible after birth. Breastfeed frequently to avoid engorgement. Use nipple rolling or stretching before each breastfeeding. Pump your breast for a short period before breastfeeding, or try ice wrapped in a cloth and placed on the nipple before feeding. Breast shells (milk cups) may be used between feedings. Remove the breast shell just before placing baby at your breast.
Nipples, Rubber	Avoid rubber nipples for the first several weeks of breastfeeding. Babies may be confused by the rubber nipple and refuse to breastfeed. Pacifiers should not be used as a substitute for frequent breastfeeding.
Nipple Shields	Nipple shields are soft plastic or rubber devices designed to be placed over the human nipple. Nipple shields interfere with milk production and may result in poor weight gain in your baby. They may confuse baby on how to breastfeed. Nipple shields are not recommended (see "Rubber Nipples").
Nipples, Sore	Nipple tenderness commonly occurs, but breastfeeding should not be painful. Correct latch-on and proper positioning of baby can prevent or minimize soreness. If nipples are sore: vary baby's position on breast; air dry nipples after feeding; avoid soap, alcohol, or nipple creams; use shorter, more frequent feedings; use least sore breast first; rub a few drops of breastmilk on nipple after feeding.

Table 6.2
BREASTFEEDING TIPS Continued

Concern	Recommended Action
Plugged Duct	A plugged duct is a tender or sore lump in the breast. Common causes: tight bra; sleeping on stomach; poor positioning; delayed/infrequent breastfeeding. Feed every 2–3 hours. Apply warm, moist heat 10–15 minutes before feeding. Massage breast before and during feeding. Change baby's position each feeding. Take non-aspirin pain reliever. Untreated plugged ducts may lead to mastitis.
Position of Mother	Relax in a comfortable position with extra pillows for support. Do not lean over baby; bring baby to your breast.
Position of Baby—Cradle Hold	Hold your baby with the baby's head resting in the bend of your arm. Baby should be tummy to tummy with you. His/her face, chest, shoulder, and knees should all be facing you. Your arm should support your baby's bottom or upper thigh. Baby needs to remain at breast level.
Position of Baby—Football Hold	Support the baby by your side with one or two pillows. The baby's bottom should touch the chair or bed; his/her legs should extend upward. Your arm will support baby's back, and your hand should firmly support the base of your baby's head. Baby's mouth should be at nipple level.

Adapted with permission from Breastfeeding Helper. Copyright 1991, Nutrition Council of Arizona Breastfeeding Advocates.

Table 6.3
POSSIBLE PROBLEMATIC MEDICATIONS DURING LACTATION

Medications Contraindicated	Abuse Drugs Contraindicated	Medications to Be Given with Caution
Bromocriptine	Amphetamine	Aspirin (salicylates)
Cipro	Cocaine	Clemastine
Cocaine	Heroin	Phenobarbital
Cyclosporine	Marijuana	Primidone
Doxorubicin	Nicotine	Salicylazo-sulfapyridine (sulfasalazine)
Ergotamine	Phencyclidine	
Lithium		
Methotrexate		
Phencyclidine		
Phenindione		

Modified from Transfer of Drugs and Chemicals into Human Milk. *Copyright 1989, American Academy of Pediatrics.*

Table 6.4
FOODS AND BEVERAGES WHICH MAY CAUSE G.I. DISTRESS TO BREASTFEEDING INFANTS

Caffeine-containing foods/beverages:
  Chocolate
  Coffee
  Colas
  Teas

Cruciferous vegetables:
  Beans
  Broccoli
  Cabbage
  Cauliflower

Foods associated with allergy (if family history is positive for food allergies):
  Egg white
  Fish
  Milk
  Peanuts
  Wheat

Other:
  Fried foods
  Oils

Breastfeeding Resources

For more information on breastfeeding, contact

- Local childbirth education associations
- County health department
- Local hospitals
- La Leche League (708) 455-7730
- Medela Breastfeeding Products 1-800-435-8316

Infant Formulas

Formulas and Methods of Preparation

Table 6.5 lists four types of commonly available formula. Proper formula preparation is essential to reduce the risk for G.I. infections, improper growth velocity (inadequate or excess), constipation, or electrolyte imbalances due to improper dilution. Water, nipples, and bottles should be sterilized for the first 3–4 months.

Selection and Composition of Commercial Infant Formulas

Controversy surrounds the selection of infant formulas. The best formulas are those which most closely resemble breastmilk. Formulas can almost imitate breastmilk in protein and carbohydrate composition, but they have no living organisms, no nucleic acids, no cholesterol, no lactose, and the fat and protein sources are different. In particular, formulas have minimal (if any) omega-3 fatty acids and their protein is derived primarily from casein. Breastmilk continues to be the first, second, and third best choice. However, in cases where formula *must* be used, a wide variety of products are available. Tables 6.6 to 6.8 provide characteristics of the leading milk-based, soy-based, and special formulas.

Milk-based formulas are satisfactory for most infants. Soy-based formulas may be used for vegetarians, infants who have IgE-mediated reaction to cow's milk proteins, or infants who have lactase deficiency (soy-based formulas do not contain lactose). Minor intolerances to milk-based formulas such as colic, loose stools, spitting up, or vomiting sometimes prompt a change to soy formula. Most of these minor problems are unrelated to the feeding. Infants occasionally respond positively to soy formulas for reasons not totally understood. Infants who are intolerant to milk and soy can generally tolerate a protein hydrolysate formula or a highly digestible formula such as Pregestamil.

Table 6.5
TYPES OF FORMULAS AND METHODS OF PREPARATION

Type	Formula Description	How to Prepare
Concentrate	Liquid formula that must be mixed with water at a 1:1 ratio.	Wash the top of formula can. Shake formula can and punch two holes using a clean punch-type can opener. Add equal amounts of concentrate and water to bottle. Formula should be used within 2 days of opening.
Evaporated Milk	Canned, concentrated cow's milk. This is not an infant formula.	Add one 13-oz can of whole evaporated milk fortified with vitamins A and D to 19 oz of water; add 1 oz (2 Tbsp) of sugar. Supplement with vitamin C. NOTE: This is not a recommended formula due to inadequate vitamin supplementation.
Powdered	This is a dry formula, one level scoop to 2 oz of water (least expensive).	Add one packed level scoop of powder to each 2 oz of water in the bottle.
Ready-to-Feed	Generally comes in cans and is ready-to-serve (most expensive).	No preparation necessary. Cans should be used within 2 days of opening. Formula must be discarded if left at room temperature for more than 2 hours.

Table 6.6
COMPOSITION OF MILK-BASED FORMULAS

Nutritional Characteristics	Human milk g/dL (% kcal)	Unmodified cow's milk g/dL (% kcal)	Enfamil (M. Johnson) g/dL (% kcal)	Similac (Ross) g/dL (% kcal)	SMA (Wyeth) g/dL (% kcal)
Energy	20 kcal/oz	20 kcal/oz	20 kcal/oz	20 kcal/oz	20 kcal/oz
Carbohydrate	7.2 (38)	4.8 (29)	7.0 (41)	7.2 (43)	7.2 (41)
Carbohydrate Source	Lactose	Lactose	Lactose	Lactose	Lactose
Fat	3.6 (56)	3.7 (50)	3.8 (50)	3.7 (48)	3.6 (50)
Fat Source	Human fat	Butterfat	Coconut oil Soy oil Palm oil Sunlower oil	Coconut oil Soy oil	Oleo, coconut, safflower oil, and soybean oil
Protein	1.1 (6)	3.3 (21)	1.5 (9)	1.5 (9)	1.5 (9)
Protein Source	Human milk proteins	Butterfat	Non-fat milk with whey added	Non-fat milk	Non-fat milk with whey added
Whey Casein	60:40	18:82	60:40	18:82	60:40

Table 6.7
COMPOSITION OF SOY-BASED FORMULAS

Nutritional Characteristics	Nursoy (Wyeth) g/dL (% kcal)	Isomil (Ross) g/dL (% kcal)	ProSobee (M. Johnson) g/dL (% kcal)	Alsoy (carnation) g/dL (% kcal)
Energy	20 kcal/oz	20 kcal/oz	20 kcal/oz	20 kcal/oz
Carbohydrate	6.9 (40)	6.8 (40)	6.8 (40)	6.7 (39)
Carbohydrate Source	Sucrose (liquid) corn syrup solids and sucrose (powder)	Corn syrup solids, sucrose	Corn syrup solids	Sucrose, tapioca, starch, and dextrins (concentrate potato, maltodextran (powder)
Fat	3.6 (47)	3.7 (49)	3.6 (48)	3.8 (49)
Fat Source	Oleo, coconut, safflower oil, and soybean oil	Soybean Coconut	Palmolein, soy, coconut, and high oleic safflower oil	Soy oil
Protein	1.8 (13)	1.8 (11)	2.0 (12)	2.1 (12)
Protein Source	Soy protein isolates plus L-methionine, L-carnitine, and	Soy protein isolates plus L-methionine, L-carnitine, and	Soy protein isolates plus L-methionine, L-carnitine, and	Soy protein isolates, L-methionine, L-carnitine, and

Table 6.8
COMPOSITION OF SPECIAL USE INFANT FORMULAS

Nutritional Characteristics	Nutramigen g/dL (% kcal)	Pregestamil g/dL (% kcal)	Pediasure g/dL (% kcal)	Lactofree g/dL (% kcal)	Similac Special Care g/dL (% kcal)
Energy	20 kcal/oz	20 kcal/oz	30 kcal/oz	20 kcal/oz	20 kcal/oz
Carbohydrate	7.4 (44)	10.3 (40)	10.9 (44)	7 (41)	8.6 (42)
Carbohydrate Source	Corn starch and corn syrup solids	Corn syrup solids, glucose, cornstarch	Hydrolyzed cornstarch and sucrose	Glucose polymers from corn syrup	Hydrolyzed corn starch, lactose
Fat	3.4 (45)	3.8 (50)	4.9 (44)	3.8 (50)	4.4 (49)
Fat Source	Soy oil, Palm oil, Coconut oil, Sunflower oil	Corn oil, MCT, high oleic safflower oil, and soy oil	MCT, safflower oil, and soy oil	Palm oil, Sunflower oil, Coconut, and Soy oil	MCT oil, Soy oil, Coconut oil
Protein	2.0 (11)	1.9 (11)	3.0 (12)	1.5 (9)	2.0 (10)
Protein Source	Casein hydrolysates	Casein hydrolysates	Casein hydrolysates, whey	Skim milk and whey	Skim milk and whey

Information collected from manufacturers, 1995.

Altering Energy Intake

Occasionally, clinicians will want to prescribe a diluted formula (to reduce hypertonic diarrhea, increase fluid intake) or a concentrated formula (to promote weight gain or increase energy intake). Tables 6.9 through 6.12 provide information regarding energy density of standard infant formulas, as well as methods for altering the caloric concentration of food and formulas to achieve the desired outcomes.

Table 6.9
INCREASING ENERGY INTAKE FOR WEIGHT GAIN IN INFANTS

- Provide food every 2-3 hours, but not more often than every hour.
- Increase energy content of formula (see Tables 6.10, 6.11, and 6.12).
- Add margarine or butter to solid foods.
- Choose high energy concentration foods (see Table 2.12).
- Make sure meal times are consistent, structured, and fun.

Table 6.10
ALTERING ENERGY CONCENTRATIONS OF LIQUID FORMULAS

	Liquid Formula Concentrate (fl oz)	Water (fl oz)	Final Volume (fl oz)
10	2	6	8
15	3	5	8
20*	4	4	8
24**	4.8	3.2	8
27**	5.4	2.6	8
30**	6	2	8

* *The standard concentration of ready-made formula is 20 kcal/oz. Currently marketed formula concentrates that require only the addition of water are 40 kcal/oz before dilution.*

***Note: Higher caloric concentration indicates higher osmolality, which can precipitate diarrhea and dehydration.*

Table 6.11
ALTERING ENERGY CONCENTRATIONS OF POWDERED FORMULAS

Desired Energy Concentration (kcal/oz)	Powdered Formula (1 oz = 1 scoop)	Water (oz)	Final Volume (fl oz)
10	2	8	8.2
15	3	8	8.5
20*	4	8	8.8
24**	4.8	7	8
28**	5.6	7	8.5

* *The standard concentration of ready-made formula is 20 kcal/oz. Powdered infant formulas are 40 kcal/Tbsp (level, packed). For large volumes of formula, because the powder displaces the water and makes the volume larger and the formula more dilute, water should be added to the powder to equal the volume expected. For example, to make 32 oz of formula at 24 kcal/oz, mix 19 Tbsp with enough water (29 oz) to equal 32 oz.*

***Note: Higher caloric concentration indicates higher osmolality, which can precipitate diarrhea and dehydration.*

Table 6.12
INCREASING ENERGY CONCENTRATIONS OF INFANT FORMULAS

Additive	Amount		Final Energy Content per Ounce
Corn syrup	1 tsp		22.5 kcal
	2 tsp		25.0 kcal
	3 tsp	To	27.5 kcal
Liquid oil	1 tsp	1 cup	25.0 kcal
	2 tsp	of	30.0 kcal
	3 tsp	formula	35.0 kcal
Skim milk	1 Tbsp	at normal	23.3 kcal
powder*	2 Tbsp	concentration	26.6 kcal
Polycose®	1 Tbsp		23.8 kcal
	2 Tbsp		27.5 Kcal

* *1 tbsp skim milk powder will increase protein content by 0.33 gms/oz.*
Note: Higher caloric concentration indicates higher osmolality, which can precipitate diarrhea and dehydration.

Introducing Solid Foods

Guidelines for Introducing Solid Foods

Table 6.13 provides a timeline for introducing solid foods into an infant's diet.
- Introduce new foods one at a time, allowing at least a week between each new food to evaluate tolerance and potential allergy.
- Start with about 1/4 cup of the new food just once or twice a day, increase the amount little by little each day.
- If a particular food seems to cause a reaction (i.e., wheezing, rash, sore bottom) eliminate that food for 1 week, then try again. If the food has the same effect two or three times, discontinue it for at least 6 months.

Table 6.13
STEPS FOR INTRODUCING SOLID FOODS

Age of Child (mos)	Type of Solid Food	Examples of Solid Foods
5–6	Strained	Enriched cereal; strained fruits, juices, vegetables.
6–7	Mashed	By 7 months, cooked or canned fruits and vegetables, ripe banana. Teething biscuit.
7–9*	Minced fine	By 9 months, enriched bread, toast, potato, rice, macaroni. Begin finger foods, including meats.
9–12	Chopped	By 12 months, whole grain bread, cereal, bread sticks, crackers, hard cheese, pieces of fruit and vegetables, whole milk. More varied finger foods. Whole eggs (many clinicians recommend waiting until after the age of 1 year to give eggs as they can be a common cause of food allergy).
12–15	Cut table food	Begin raw fruits and vegetables.

*When introduction of increase in texture is delayed beyond this age, infant may resist change.
Note: Avoid items with added sugar and salt; encourage high-iron foods.
Reprinted with permission from "Steps in Textures" The Children's Hospital, Boston, MA, 1991.

Guidelines to Reduce Risk of Choking

Young children are at high risk of choking on food and remain at high risk until they can chew their food thoroughly ($\approx$ age 5). Remind parents that choking kills more young children then any other home accident. Table 6.14 provides guidelines to reduce choking risk.

Making Eating Safer for Young Children

1. Children should be monitored during meals and snacks to make sure they
   - Limit activity
   - Eat slowly
   - Consume only a small amount in any given spoonful or mouthful
   - Chew food well before swallowing

Table 6.14
FOODS THAT CAN CAUSE CHOKING IN CHILDREN UNTIL AGE 5

- Firm, smooth, or slippery foods which can slide down the throat before chewing, such as
    - grapes
    - hot dogs
    - hard candy
    - lollipops
    - peanuts
- Small, dry, or hard foods that are difficult to chew and easy to swallow whole, such as
    - French fries
    - popcorn
    - potato and corn chips
    - nuts and seeds
    - small pieces of raw carrots
- Sticky or tough foods that do not break apart easily and are hard to remove from the airways, such as
    - peanut butter
    - raisins and other dried fruit
    - tough meat

Adapted from "Nutrition Update: Preventing Young Children from Choking on Food," Number 2, Food and Consumer Service, Nutrition and Technical Services Division, Nutrition Science and Education Branch, Alexandria, Virginia, © 1988.

2. Table foods should be prepared so they are easy to chew:
   - Grind up tough foods
   - Cut food into small pieces or thin slices
   - Cut round foods, like hot dogs, into short strips rather than round pieces
   - Take out all bones from fish, chicken, and meat
   - Take out seeds and pits from fruits
3. Other foods that may cause allergic reactions or gastrointestinal upset should be avoided (see Table 6.15).

Promoting Healthy Teeth

Teeth and gum care is important during infancy and childhood. Table 6.16 provides teeth and gum care guidelines to promote healthy dentition.

Teething Tips

During teething, babies may drool, be fussy, and have diarrhea, fever, and changes in appetite. Advise mothers to
- Gently rub baby's gums with clean finger.
- Offer a cold, hard rubber teething ring, ice wrapped in a clean towel, or a clean, frozen face cloth. DO NOT leave baby alone with ice because of choking risk.
- Use teething medication sparingly.

Proper Bottle Use Advice

- Provide only expressed breastmilk, formula, or plain water from a bottle.
- Use the bottle only for feeding. A bottle is not a pacifier or toy.
- The sugar found in formula, milk, juice, and sweetened drinks can decay the teeth.
- Sleeping times are not feeding times. Do not put baby to bed with a bottle. This can cause ear infections and tooth decay called "Nursing Bottle Mouth."
- Use comfort techniques such as offering a blanket, stuffed animal, or favorite toy instead of a bottle.

Feeding Toddlers and Young Children

Many toddlers and young children use food to assert their independence. Table 6.17 provides practical interventions for dealing with unhealthy power struggles associated with food.

Table 6.15
FOODS NOT TO FEED TO INFANTS

Home-Prepared Baby Foods	Foods That May Cause Choking	Allergy-Related Foods	Difficult to Digest Foods
Canned vegetables or preseasoned family foods, because of the high sodium content. Home-prepared, vegetables high in nitrate such as beets, spinach, turnips, mustard, and collard greens.	Candies Celery Cookies Corn Fruits with seeds Hot dogs Nuts, peanuts Popcorn Potato chips Raisins	Chocolate Citrus Cocoa Egg whites Milk Peanuts Tomatoes Wheat	Bacon Fatty foods Fried foods Highly spiced foods Sausage Whole-kernel corn

IMPORTANT:
- Never introduce cow's milk earlier than 6 months of age. It may cause G.I. blood loss and/or iron deficiency.
- Honey introduced during infancy has been associated with botulism poisoning. Honey should NOT be given to children under 1 year of age.

Reprinted with permission from: Austin C. "Dietary Assessment and Management of the Infant (Birth through Two Years)," in MD Simko, C Cowell and MS Hreka,, eds. Practical Nutrition: A Quick Reference for the Health Care Practitioner, A.S.P.E.N. Publishers, Inc. 1989.

Table 6.16
TEETH AND GUM CARE GUIDELINES

Age of Child	Care Instructions
Birth–1 year	Wipe baby's gums and teeth with a clean, wet cloth or gauze daily.
1–2 years	Gently brush child's teeth with a soft toothbrush and small amount of fluoride paste daily.
2–3 years	Brush child's teeth daily. Begin to teach child to brush teeth. Take child for the first dental visit.
3–6 years	Help child brush and floss teeth daily. Take child to dentist every 6 months.
6 years and older	Remind child to brush and floss teeth daily. Encourage child to brush after eating sweet or sticky foods. Take child to dentist every 6 months.

Adapted with permission from: Massachusetts WIC Program, Department of Public Health, Boston, MA.

Table 6.18 provides ideas for balanced meals and snacks and Table 6.19 provides suggestions for healthy snacking for young children.

Increasing Energy Intake for Young Children

Some children will exhibit inadequate weight gain. The following suggestions and tables provide recommendations to promote increased weight gain.

- Make sure the child has regular meal and snack times. Recommend 3 meals and 3 snacks a day (breakfast, snack, lunch, snack, dinner, snack).
- Provide child with high-calorie drinks like milkshakes, instant breakfast, Pediasure®.
- Increase calories by "Power Packing" foods as much as possible. This way the child gets a lot of calories in each small bite.

Table 6.17 provides suggestions for making foods calorically dense.

Table 6.17
INCREASING ENERGY INTAKE FOR WEIGHT GAIN IN YOUNG CHILDREN

To these foods:	Add these ingredients:
bread, tortillas, crackers, potatoes, rice, vegetables, beans	cheese, cream cheese, sour cream
bread, tortillas, crackers, apples, bananas, celery, carrots	peanut butter, nuts (NOTE: Not recommended for children younger than 36 months)
bread, tortillas, crackers, potatoes, rice, cooked vegetables, cereal	margarine, butter
cereal, salad, fruit, ice cream, yogurt	raisins, prunes, dates
milk	instant breakfast
milk, cereal, waffles, pancakes	syrup, sugar, drink mixes
milk, cereal, pudding, potatoes, soups, scrambled eggs, noodles, pasta	cream, half-and-half, cheese
potatoes, vegetables, noodles	salad dressing, white sauces, cheese
puddings, yogurt, ice cream, pureed fruit	crushed graham crackers
puddings, yogurt, casseroles, soups	powdered milk, margarine, butter, cheese
puddings, ice cream, fruit, cooked cereal	whipped cream
tortillas, crackers, sandwiches, beans, salads, vegetables	avocado
vegetables, sandwiches	mayonnaise, cheese
yogurt, fruit, ice cream, cream	granola (NOTE: Not recommended for children younger than 24 months) oil (gradually work up to 1 Tbsp per 8 oz milk/yogurt)

Table 6.18
CHILDHOOD FEEDING PROBLEMS AND SOLUTIONS

Problem	Suggested Solution
Refuses to eat altogether	• Eating jags are very common, especially in preschool children. Appetite changes account for much of the variation and the eat-then-don't-eat pattern, due to physiological changes in metabolism, activity, and growth; provide a variety of foods, as well as preferred foods. • Children are also wary of new or combination foods. A child is likely to reject a new food simply because it is unfamiliar. Involving children in meal preparation and serving familiar foods more frequently decreases food battles. • A well-nourished child who suddenly decides to eat only one or two foods will entually become bored with them and start eating after a week or two. It is especially important that the parents do not make a big deal of it. • Children that refuse to eat so much that they lose weight need to be evaluated for an underlying medical condition and/or family or individual problems.
Asserting independence	• A reason for refusing to eating certain foods is that children use food fights to test their power within the family. The food itself is largely irrelevant. The child sees it as a way of asserting his/her independence. • Offering the child choices helps to provide other less difficult ways of asserting independence, such as: "Do you want the white cup or the blue cup?" "Do you want milk or juice?", etc.

continued on next page

Table 6.18
CHILDHOOD FEEDING PROBLEMS AND SOLUTIONS *Continued*

Problem	Suggested Solution
Sweets, eats too many	• Eliminate from home. • Use "natural" sweets such as fruits. • Avoid using sweets as a reward or bribe. • Provide exciting alternatives, i.e., pizza bagels or apple faces. • Provide cookies, with added fruit. • Provide fruitshakes.
Breads and cereals, refuses	• Serve cooked cereal warm, not hot. • Add raisins or fresh fruit to cereal. • Add yogurt or fruit to cereal. • Offer toast instead of bread (cut in small pieces). Offer tortillas and pasta. • Use fruit spreads on bread.
Fruits and/or vegetables, refuses	• If refuses vegetables, offer more fruits. • Without forcing, slowly introduce small portions of vegetables (raw bite-sized pieces; vegetables cooked crisp rather than overcooked). • Children learn from their parents' examples; when parents eat vegetables, children are more likely to try them as well. • Young children are capable of detecting flavors that their parents cannot, especially bitter flavors in certain vegetables. • Serve raw fruits or vegetables with dips. • Add grated vegetables or fruit to recipes. • Offer blenderized drinks with fruit, i.e., bananas and strawberries.
Meat, refuses	• Mince or grind; provide bite size pieces of moist meat or meat that is easy to chew. Offer other protein sources, i.e., peanut butter, beans, cheese, tofu, and textured vegetable protein. • Serve with gravy, catsup, or barbecue sauce.

Table 6.18
CHILDHOOD FEEDING PROBLEMS AND SOLUTIONS *Continued*

Problem	Suggested Solution
Milk, refuses	• Serve at room temperature (cold milk may be painful to a teething child). • Let child pour from a small pitcher or sip through a colored straw. • Cook cereals with milk; offer creamed soups and milk desserts. • Offer cheese and yogurt; add powdered milk to recipes. • Use flavorings.
Milk, drinks too much	• Offer milk after meals only. • Offer water if thirsty between meals. • Offer milk in smaller containers.

Adapted with permission from "Feeding Solutions" The Children's Hospital, Boston, MA. 1991.

Table 6.19
IDEAS FOR BALANCED MEALS AND SNACKS

BREAKFAST (Choose at least 1 food from each group)
1. Main course
   - Pancakes, waffles, French toast with syrup and margarine
   - Oatmeal, Malt-O-Meal, cream of wheat with sugar or syrup and margarine
   - Scrambled eggs with cheese, tortillas
   - Bagels or toast with cream cheese or cheese
   - Chorizo and eggs, tortillas
   - Dry cereal or cereal with milk or yogurt
2. Fruit
   - Banana
   - Orange slices
   - Apple slices
   - Other seasonal fruits
3. Drink
   - Milk or fruit juice

continued on next page

Table 6.19
IDEAS FOR BALANCED MEALS AND SNACKS *Continued*

SNACK (Choose at least 2 foods from 2 different groups)
Provide in between meals so that food is offered every 2–3 hours.

1. Main course
   - Crackers, graham crackers
   - Cookies, tortillas, bread
   - Dry cereal
2. Side dish
   - Nuts, peanut butter
   - Cheese, cream cheese, cottage cheese
   - Dressing for vegetables
3. Fruit/Vegetable
   - Fresh fruit
   - Raisins, prunes, dates
   - Canned fruit
   - Cut up vegetables
   - Avocados
4. Drink
   - Fruit juice or milk

LUNCH (Choose at least 1 food from each group)

1. Main course
   - Spaghetti, Spaghetti-O's, macaroni and cheese, noodles with cream or sauce
   - Sandwich with mayonnaise and meat or cheese, or peanut butter and jelly
   - Tortillas and cheese and/or beans
   - Bread and cheese
   - Soup
   - Casseroles or tacos, enchiladas, tamales
   - Meat, fish, poultry
2. Fruits/Vegetables
   - Peas, corn, beans
   - Potatoes, sweet potatoes, rice
   - Apples, bananas, oranges, grapes, cantaloupe, watermelon
   - Canned peaches, pears, pineapple, fruit cocktail
   - Carrots, broccoli, cauliflower, zucchini, green beans
   - Other fruits and vegetables in season

continued on next page

Table 6.19
IDEAS FOR BALANCED MEALS AND SNACKS *Continued*

LUNCH *Continued*

3. Starch
   - Noodles, pasta
   - Bread, rolls
   - Tortillas, crackers, chips
4. Drink
   - Milk or fruit juice
5. Optional
   - Pudding, fruit yogurt
   - Cookies, cake
   - Ice cream, popsicles

DINNER (Choose at least 1 food from each group)

1. Main course
   - Spaghetti, Spaghetti-O's, macaroni and cheese, noodles with cream or sauce
   - Sandwich with mayonnaise and meat or cheese, or peanut butter and jelly
   - Tortillas and cheese and/or beans
   - Bread and cheese
   - Soup
   - Casseroles or tacos, enchiladas, tamales
   - Meat, fish, poultry
2. Side dish
   - Peas, corn, beans
   - Potatoes, sweet potatoes, rice
   - Noodles, pasta
   - Bread, rolls
3. Fruits/Vegetables
   - Apples, bananas, oranges, grapes, cantaloupe, watermelon
   - Canned peaches, pears, pineapple, fruit cocktail
   - Carrots, broccoli, cauliflower, zucchini, green beans
   - Other fruits and vegetables in season
4. Drink
   - Milk or fruit juice
5. Optional
   - Pudding, fruit yogurt
   - Cookies, cake
   - Ice cream, popsicles

Table 6.20
HEALTHY SNACKS FOR YOUNG CHILDREN

Choose More Often	Choose Less Often
• Cereal, unsweetened • Dried fruits • Fresh fruit • Frozen fruit popsicles • Frozen yogurt, low-fat • Fruit juice, unsweetened • Low fat cookies such as vanilla wafers, animals or graham crackers • Pretzels	• Candy • Cheese, regular cottage cheese • Chips • High fat cookies such as chocolate, iced or icing-filled • Ice cream or candy-coated popsicles • Peanut butter • Soda pop

Feeding School-Age and Adolescent Children

As children enter school, their nutritional needs and issues may change. (See Table 1.6) Additionally, efforts should be made to optimize the child's diet to reduce risk for chronic disease.

Dietary Fat

The relationships between a high-fat diet, obesity, and heart disease are now well proven. Studies also suggest that a high-fat diet can contribute to certain kinds of cancer. Groups such as the National Heart Lung and Blood Institute have recommended that children's diet not exceed a fat level greater than 30% of calories. The average diet currently obtains 34% of calories from fat. Table 6.21 provides some recommendations to parents for reducing fat (see also Healthy snacks for young children, Table 6.20).

Table 6.21
REDUCING FAT INTAKE IN SCHOOL-AGE AND ADOLESCENT CHILDREN

- Balance diets. Pizza one day; skinless chicken the next.
- Keep high-fat foods off the table; for instance, spread margarine thinly on bread before serving.
- Pay attention to recommended serving sizes, especially meats and poultry.
- Keep nutritious snacks on hand, including fruit, cold cereal, low-fat yogurt, frozen fruit popsicles, and low-fat crackers. (See Table 6.20)
- Do not force kids to clean their plates.
- Never deep fry. Use monounsaturated oil for cooking.
- Choose the lowest-fat alternative at fast-food restaurants.
- Eating right is a family affair. Children will eat healthy foods if their parents do.

Factors Associated with Nutritional Risk

Characteristics of children with higher nutritional risk factors include:
- Children from deprived families, especially those who are abused or neglected.
- Children with poor appetites, and poor eating habits.
- Children consuming vegetarian diets without dairy products.
- Children with chronic illness, especially those requiring special diets. See also page 35.

Importance of Breakfast/School Feeding

Many children do not eat breakfast or have well-balanced meals. Figure 6.2 illustrates the importance of breakfast for improving energy levels in the morning.

Sports Nutrition

Good nutrition along with training, natural ability, skill, and motivation are the major factors that influence performance. There are no "magic" foods that will produce super stars.

What Should Athletes Eat?
- Keep food intake regular; do not skip meals.
- Forget the fads; select meals from the Food Guide Pyramid.
- Select complex carbohydrates such as breads, cereal, crackers, and pasta.
- Eat enough to maintain body weight; avoid drastic weight changes.

Weight Control
- Crash diets can lower energy reserves.
- Drying out for early weigh-ins can lead to severe dehydration and poor performance.
- Maintain body weight by regular food and fluid intake.

Pregame Meals
- Avoid overeating before competition.
- Eat complex carbohydrates 3-4 hours before the event or competition. Examples are pasta, rice, bread, potatoes, grains, and legumes.
- Drink water before and during competition.

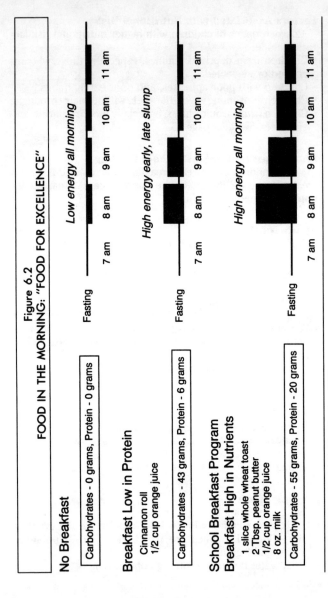

Eating for All-Day Sporting Events

All-day events such as running, swimming, tennis, and gymnastics require a lot of energy and a steady supply of nutrients. The following guideline lists when and what to eat during competition intervals.

One hour or less before competition
- Fruit and vegetable juices such as orange, tomato, or V-8 juices and/or
- Fresh fruit such as watermelon, peaches, grapes, or oranges

Two to three hours before competition
- Fruit juices and fresh fruit and/or
- Breads, bagels, or muffins, with a limited amount of butter or cream cheese

Three to four hours before competition
- Fruit juices and fresh fruit and
- Breads, bagels, or muffins and
- A light spread of peanut butter or slice of cheese for breads, or a light spread of cream cheese for bagels and/or
- Bowl of cereal with low-fat milk

Four hours or more
- Sandwich with 2 slices of bread and 2 oz of lean meat and
- Fresh fruit and
- Fresh vegetables and
- Low-fat milk

Convenient Snacks for the Athlete
- Breads, bagels, muffins
- Crackers, pretzels
- Dried fruits
- Fig newtons, oatmeal cookies, raisin cookies
- Fresh fruits and vegetables
- Fruit juices, or tomato or V-8 juices
- Individual boxes of breakfast cereal

Water Requirements

Water is the most important nutrient for the athlete and is the preferred choice for fluid replacement. Dehydration, heat stroke, organ damage, and possible death might result if water is withheld.
- 1–2 cups 5–15 minutes before a workout or competition
- 8–10 oz every 15–20 minutes of strenuous exercise

Vitamin/Mineral Supplementation

The American Academy of Pediatrics does not recommend routine vitamin/mineral supplementation for healthy children, except for fluoride supplementation in areas where the water is unfluoridated. However, the following population groups are at higher nutritional risk and could potentially benefit from routine supplementation with a multivitamin/mineral to provide the level of nutrients in the RDA (see Table 1.2).

- Physically active people have higher caloric intakes and therefore obtain additional vitamins from their diets. Low-dose vitamin C supplementation may help endurance athletes (see Tables 1.2 and 1.3).
- Athletic training increases **calcium** demand beyond that needed for growth alone. Calcium-containing foods and/or supplements need to be consumed to provide 1000 mg daily (see Table 2.1).
- Insufficient **iron** in the blood can impair physical performance. Adolescents have higher iron demands of rapidly growing muscles. Adolescent endurance athletes are at higher risk of iron-deficiency anemia. Encourage iron-rich foods (see Table 2.3) and monitor status when indicated (see Table 4.7).
- Sodium losses in perspiration can be sustained, although losses decrease as fitness increases. Losses can be easily replaced by a normal diet.

SECTION 7
Disease-Specific Feeding Issues

Disease-Specific Feeding Issues

Several disease- or health-related concerns can arise throughout infancy and childhood. The following section provides practical guidelines for nutritional intervention specific to the health problem encountered.

Table 7.1
COMMON DIET-RELATED PROBLEMS

Problem	Causes	Counseling
Colic or colicky symptoms	• Food intolerance • Improper feeding techniques • Inadequate breastmilk • Overfeeding with formula • Unknown cause	• Counsel on comfort techniques and interpreting hunger cues. • Eliminate possible offending foods. • Feeding techniques: small, frequent meals, proper position, more burping. • Pleasant environment. • Breastmilk increased by increased offering, longer sucking.
Constipation	• Exercise • Fiber • Inadequate fluids	• Increase fluids (see Table 3.1). • Add fruit juice (i.e., grape, apple). • Decrease solids if introduction too rapid (infants). • Add bulk (whole grains, bran, fresh fruits, vegetables, legumes) (see Table 2.2). • Increase activity.
Diarrhea	• **Acute:** Gastro-enteritis • **Chronic:** Poor treatment of acute diarrhea, food intolerance, or allergy	• Maintain fluid and electrolyte balance. Continue breastfeeding or oral rehydration solution (i.e., Pedialyte) for 24 hours (see Table 3.1). • Reintroduce solids after 24 hours. Initial food should include diluted formula, rice cereal, bananas, and potatoes. • Omit offending food, discontinue pear and apple, fruit juices, or other highly sweetened beverages.

Table 7.1
COMMON DIET-RELATED PROBLEMS *Continued*

Problem	Causes	Counseling
Food allergy or intolerance	Most common food allergens include • cow's milk • wheat • egg whites • corn • citrus • peanuts	• Eliminate and then challenge with the offending food. • Check for symptoms to confirm diagnosis. • See Tables 7.11, 7.12, and 7.13.
Refusal to eat	• Unknown cause • Improper feeding techniques • Inadequate response to infant cues • Organic illness	• Consistent, calm, structured provision of food. • Pay attention to infant body language. • Consider illness as cause if other symptoms are present.
Regurgitation	• G.I. reflux • Immature gut • Improper feeding technique	• Semisitting feeding position. • Frequent upright burping. • No large nipple holes. • Gentle handling.
Vomiting	• Gastroenteritis • Food borne illness • Food intolerance	• Omit one to two feeds. • Maintain fluid and electrolyte balance (Table 3.1). • Continue breastfeeding. • Reintroduce solids after 24 hours. • Initial foods should include diluted formula, rice cereal, bananas, potatoes, and other non-lactose carbohydrate-rich foods.

Cardiovascular Disease

Screening Recommendations

Cholesterol testing is recommended for children whose parents or grandparents had:
- Documented myocardial infarction, positive coronary angiogram, cerebrovascular disease, or peripheral vascular disease before age 55, or
- A serum cholesterol level of 240 mg/dL or greater.

Table 7.2
EVALUATION OF SERUM CHOLESTEROL LEVELS

Category	Total Cholesterol (mg/dL)	LDL Cholesterol (mg/dL)
Acceptable	<170	<110
Borderline	170–199	110–129
High	>200	>130

Adapted with permission from Highlights of the Report of the Expert Panel on Blood Cholesterol Levels in Children & Adolescents. Pediatrics 89(3):525–584, 1992.

Table 7.3
CURRENT VS. RECOMMENDED FAT INTAKE IN CHILDREN AND ADOLESCENTS WITH CVD

Type of Fat	Current Intake*	Recommended Intake
Total fat, % of calories	35–36	Average no more than 30
Saturated fatty acids, %	14	<10
Polyunsaturated, %	6	Up to 10
Monounsaturated, %	13–14	10–15
Cholesterol, mg/day	193–296	<300

*Preliminary data from U.S. Department of Agriculture's 1987-1988 Nationwide Food Consumption Survey.

Adapted with permission from Highlights of the Report of the Expert Panel on Blood Cholesterol Levels in Children & Adolescents. Pediatrics 89(3):525–584, 1992.

Dietary Intervention for the Prevention and Treatment of Cardiovascular Disease*

Table 7.4
RECOMMENDED INTAKES ON THE STEP-ONE AND STEP-TWO DIETS FOR CARDIOVASCULAR DISEASE

Nutrient	Step-One Diet	Step-Two Diet
Calories	To promote normal growth and development and to reach or maintain desirable body weight	Same as Step-One Diet
Carbohydrates	About 55% of total calories	Same as Step-One
Cholesterol	Less than 300 mg/day	Less than 200 mg/day
Fatty acids		
Monounsaturated =	Remaining total fat calories	Same as Step-One
Polyunsaturated =	Up to 10% of total calories	Same as Step-One
Saturated =	Less than 10% of total calories	Less than 7% of total calories
Protein	About 15–20% of total calories	Same as Step-One
Total fat	Average of no more than 30% of total calories	Same as Step-One

*Children under 2 years of age should not have dietary fat or cholesterol restricted at any level.

Adapted with permission from Highlights of the Report of the Expert Panel on Blood Cholesterol in Children and Adolescents. Pediatrics 89(3): 525–584, 1992.

Table 7.5
DIET THERAPY VS. DRUG THERAPY
IN CARDIOVASCULAR DISEASE TREATMENT

Diet Therapy

Diet therapy is the primary approach to treating children and adolescents. The goals of diet therapy are as follows:

1. For borderline LDL cholesterol:
   - To lower the level to <110 mg/dL.

2. For high LDL cholesterol:
   - To lower the level to <130 mg/dL as a minimal goal.
   - To lower the level to <110 mg/dL as an ideal goal.

Drug Therapy

Consider drug therapy in children 10 years of age or older if, after an adequate trial of diet therapy (6 months to 1 year):

1. LDL cholesterol remains ≥ 190 mg/dL: *or*

2. LDL cholesterol remains >160 mg/dL *and*
   - There is a positive family history of premature CVD (<55 years).
   - Two or more other CVD risk factors are present after vigorous attempts have been made to control these risk factors.

NOTE: Although no specific recommendations have been developed there is accumulating evidence that antioxidant nutrients (vitamins A, C, and E, beta-carotenoids, riboflavin, selenium, manganese, zinc, and copper) play a key role in reducing the risk of heart disease. This means eat more whole grains, fruits, and vegetables at least until more specific recommendations are available.

Adapted from Highlights of the Report of the Expert Panel on Blood Cholesterol Levels in Children and Adolescents. Pediatrics 89(3):S25–S84, 1992.

Eating Disorders

General Information

The term "eating disorder" includes anorexia nervosa, bulimia nervosa, any combination of the two, or eating disorder not otherwise specified. Individualized nutrition recommendations are based on a nutritional assessment which includes anthropometric data, biochemical data, dietary history, behavioral history, exercise history, and information obtained from a psychological evaluation. Due to the complexity of eating disorders, a team approach is used. The team consists, at a minimum, of a psychologist/psychiatrist, a registered dietitian, and a medical doctor.

Common eating disorder profiles include easy filling/bloating, eating slowly, eating alone, preoccupation with food, fear of loss of control when they begin to eat, knowledge of caloric content of food, use of large amounts of condiments, binge eating with or without fasting or purging, aversion to particular foods or groups of foods, and eating an inadequate quantity of an acceptable variety of foods.

Currently 0.5% of females have been clinically diagnosed with anorexia nervosa and 1-3% with bulimia nervosa. Subclinical eating disorders occur in 3-5% of the female population in the United States. Prevention of eating disorders is an area of active research. Risk factors have been identified, but interventions to prevent these diseases have not been empirically validated.

Suggestions Which May Help Reduce Risk for Developing an Eating Disorder

- Discourage dieting/dieting behaviors in young females.
- Encourage consumption of a well-balanced diet that includes a variety of foods.
- Provide support to females during critical transition periods such as puberty, change in schools or family status, etc.
- Monitor for other high-risk behaviors which tend to occur concurrent with eating disorders, such as unsafe sexual practices, and drug and/or alcohol abuse.

Recommended Treatment/Intervention for Eating Disorders

- Make an individualized treatment plan.
- Education includes teaching the patient about individual

nutrient needs, the principles of good nutrition, the relationship between dieting and binging or starvation, establishing a pattern of healthy eating, and meal planning by using a food exchange system.
- Meaningful psychological and nutritional therapy is difficult to absorb and comprehend when clients are actively starving, purging, or binge eating.
- The many food-related problems surrounding eating disorders may prevent adequate qualitative and quantitative nutritional intake, so nutritional supplementa-tion is required.

Anorexia Nervosa

Signs to Look For
- Unexplained weight loss which continues beyond healthy levels.
- Complaints of constipation.
- Complaints of abdominal bloating—often receiving extensive G.I. workup.
- Orthostatic changes.
- Hypothermia.
- Bradycardia.
- Lanugo.
- Edema.
- Amenorrhea.

Nutritional Therapy
- Cessation of weight loss.
- Initiation of small frequent feedings.
- Discussion of the individual's nutrient and energy needs.
- Increasing intake dietary fiber.
- Use of a multivitamin/mineral supplement.
- Caloric progression usually starts at 800 calories (or equal to the patient's current intake) and is increased by 100 calories per day as tolerated.
- Weight gain expectations are 3/4 pound every 3 days.

Table 7.6 provides suggestions for healthy eating patterns in anorexia nervosa.

Table 7.6
HEALTHY EATING PATTERNS IN ANOREXIA NERVOSA

- Eat 6 small meals each day.
- Eat all meals and snacks sitting at a table.
- Plan meals ahead using the food exchange system.
- Eat a variety of foods from the Food Guide Pyramid (see Figure 1.1).
- Eat generous portions of foods containing complex carbohydrates, focusing on high-fiber grains.
- Limit consumption of fruits and vegetables, because they slow stomach emptying and increase the feeling of bloating.
- Gradually increase the amount of fat in the diet to meet nutritional needs.
- Avoid "trigger foods" that you associate with a binge. These can be re-introduced later.
- Limit caffeine intake, because it can reduce appetite.
- Provide a multivitamin/mineral supplement that supplies 100–150% RDA.

Developed by Adamowicz, N., and Leonard-Green, T.K. Department of Family and Community Medicine, University of Arizona (Revised 1995).

Bulimia Nervosa

Signs to Look For
- Complaints of lethargy, bloating, or constipation.
- Frequent weight fluctuations.
- Dental problems or parotid enlargement.
- Menstrual irregularities.
- Electrolyte imbalances.
- Calluses on hands/fingers from inducing emesis.
- Chronic sore throat or hoarseness.

Nutritional Therapy
- Gradual elimination of the binge/purge cycle and establishment of a more normal eating pattern.
- Discussion of the myths related to food, dieting, and weight control.
- Provide a multivitamin/mineral supplement.
- Education on strategies to regulate eating behavior.

- Restricting and semistarvation can lead to episodes of binging and purging, weight loss cannot be implemented until the eating disorder team determines it to be appropriate.
- Caloric intake is set utilizing the 1990 Mifflin resting energy expenditure calculation (Table 7.7).

Table 7.7
MIFFLIN RESTING ENERGY EXPENDITURE FORMULAS

Males

REE = 10 x weight (kg) + 6.25 x height (cm) + 5 x age (yr)–5 and adjusted to maintain weight
= _____ kcals/day required

Females

REE = 10 x weight (kg) + 6.25 x height (cm)–5 x age (yr)–161 and adjusted to maintain weight
= _____ kcals/day required

Reprinted with permission from Mifflin M et al. "A new predictive equation for resting energy expenditure in healthy individuals." Am J Clin Nutr 1990; 51:241–7.

Table 7.8 provides suggestions for healthy eating patterns in bulimia nervosa.

Table 7.8
HEALTHY EATING PATTERNS IN BULIMIA NERVOSA

- Eat three planned meals plus snacks each day, or smaller but more frequent meals.
- Eat all meals and snacks sitting at a table.
- Plan meals ahead using the food exchange system.
- Eat a variety of foods from the Food Guide Pyramid (see Figure 1.1).
- Eat generous portions of foods containing complex carbohydrates, focusing on high-fiber grains.
- Include adequate fat to increase meal satiety.
- Avoid "trigger foods" that you associate with a binge. They can be reintroduced later.
- Provide a multivitamin/mineral supplement that supplies 100–150% RDA.

Developed by Adamowicz, N., and Leonard-Green, T.K. Department of Family and Community Medicine, University of Arizona (Revised 1995).

Obesity

Obesity affects as many as 5–25% of children and adolescents within the United States and the prevalence continues to increase over all ages and sexes. Methods for defining obesity in children rely on statistical comparisons of given measurement to population norms rather than an individualized "functional" assessment of the risk of adiposity-related morbidity and the likelihood of persistence of obesity into adulthood.

Nature Versus Nurture

Less than 5% of obesity is caused by neurologic lesions, endocrinopathies, and "syndromes." The vast majority of obesity in children reflects interaction of genetics with a permissive environment. Adoption studies by Albert Stunkard showed a high correlation between the adult weights of children and their biological parents and a low correlation between children and their adoptive parents, suggesting the strong influence of genetics over environment. Similarly, a Michigan study found infants with obese mothers to be significantly heavier and fatter at birth and remain heavier up to 4 years. Combined maternal and paternal obesity produces significantly higher obesity in infants and children than any other factor. Some studies suggest that obese children eat more, faster, and select a higher-fat diet.

An equivalent amount of data has found that obese children eat no more than normal weight children, but their energy expenditure is lower. Data from the National Health Examination Survey found a significant correlation between television viewing and obesity. The prevalence of obesity increased by 2% for each additional hour of television viewed. Television viewing impacts on both activity and consumption of calorically dense foods.

Treatment for Obesity

Regardless of the etiology of obesity, the treatment requires an alteration in energy balance. Energy expenditure must be higher than the intake to cause weight loss.

The goal for children is to provide a nutritionally adequate diet and slow down or eliminate weight gain but continue to provide adequate energy to promote a bone and muscle growth, thereby creating a more acceptable weight-for-height ratio.

One method of determining an energy prescription is to calculate energy required (see Table 3.2) and subtract 300-500 calories. Specific diets are difficult to follow as well as unsuccessful in promoting permanent weight changes. Lifestyle changes such as altering the fat composition of the diet and increasing activity have a greater probability of permanently altering the body fat. Any dietary change recommendations need to be instituted by the entire family—*not* only by the target patient—and must include efforts to increase physical activity.

Table 7.9 and Table 7.10 provide suggestions for reducing fat intake and altering energy expenditure, respectively. Table 6.20 lists healthy snacks.

Table 7.9
GUIDELINES FOR REDUCING ENERGY AND FAT INTAKE

Food	Suggestion
Fruits	Eat frequently. Avoid fruits canned in syrup.
Vegetables	Choose vegetables without cream or cheese sauces. Limit consumption of avocados.
Bread, Pasta, Rice, Cereals	Use tomato based sauces. Eliminate cereal and crackers with more than 2 gm fat/serving.
Milk	Use 1% or skim after age 2. Low-fat or non-fat cheese. Low-fat or non-fat frozen desserts. Low-fat or non-fat yogurt.
Protein	Choose low-fat meat, fish or poultry without the skin. Increase consumption of alternatives like dried beans and peas. Avoid fried foods. Bake, boil, or steam.
Fat	Reduce total consumption to 1 Tbsp/day. Some fat is necessary.

See also Healthy Snacks for Young Children, Table 6.20, and Reducing Fat Intake in School-Age and Adolescent Children, Table 6.21.

Table 7.10
IDEAS FOR INCREASING ENERGY EXPENDITURE

- Limit television viewing to 1 hour or less/day.
- Increase family exercise with walks, hikes, trips to playgrounds, active games (i.e., tag or hide-and-seek).
- Park car a distance from destination.
- Take the stairs.
- Participate in organized sports (i.e., soccer, swimming, basketball, tennis).
- Promote active leisure-time activities (i.e., gymnastics and dancing).
- Parent(s) role model positive attitudes toward physical activity.

NOTE: Requirements of calisthenic or enforced aerobic exercise in obese children has been found to be associated with exercise aversion later. Greatest success is with spontaneous activities, chosen by the children which are "fun" (i.e., tag, hide-and-seek, etc.).

Food Allergies

Children can experience allergies to several different foods. Tables 7.11 through 7.13 provide eating guidelines for children diagnosed with the most common food allergies—eggs, milk, and wheat.

Table 7.11
EGG-FREE DIET

Food Group	Foods TO Eat	Foods NOT to Eat
Beverages	Fruit juices, carbonated beverages, water, milk, coffee, and tea unless cleared with egg or egg shell.	Any that contains egg or albumen. Read labels.
Breads	Ry-Krisp, or any kind of cracker or bread made without added egg; rice cakes, popcorn cakes; corn or flour tortillas or tortilla chips. Read labels.	All bread rolls, muffins, biscuits, doughnuts, popovers, sweet rolls, pancakes, waffles, pretzels, and crackers made with egg. Ingredients should not contain egg, egg powder, dried egg, or albumen.
Cereals, Grains	Any cereal. Read labels. Barley, corn meal, hominy, rice, or tapioca prepared without egg.	Pastas with added egg. Read labels.
Desserts	Plain and fruit-flavored gelatins, angel and sponge cakes, fruit pies, fruit ices, mousses, cookies, frostings, cakes, puddings, dumplings, ice creams, and sherbets without egg. Read labels.	Bavarian creams, soft or stirred and baked custards, doughnuts, fritters, macaroons, angel or sponge cakes, meringues, whips.
Fruits, Vegetables	All fruits and vegetables prepared without added egg.	Any fruit or vegetable prepared or served with a sauce containing egg.

Table 7.11
EGG-FREE DIET Continued

Food Group	Foods TO Eat	Foods NOT to Eat
Meats, Poultry, Eggs, Fish, Game, Meat Alternatives	Prepared without added egg. Do not use dried or frozen egg, egg powder, or albumen. Read labels.	Any casserole, loaf, or patty containing egg; all cheeses.
Miscellaneous	All spices, nuts, olives, pickles, popcorn, salt, spices, flavoring, extracts.	Creamed and scalloped foods; foods dipped in batter using egg; prepared mixes for biscuits, cakes, cookies, doughnuts, muffins, pie crusts, and waffles if they contain egg.
Salad Dressings, Sauces, Gravies, Soups	Catsup, mustard; gravies, meat and other sauces made without egg; dressings made without egg. Read labels.	Mayonnaise, most salad dressings, alphabet and egg noodle soup, consommés, bouillon, broths, or any soup cleared with egg. Read labels.
Sugar and Sweets	Brown, granulated, powdered, and maple sugars; honey, molasses, jellies, jams, preserves, marmalades; candies made without egg. Read labels.	Divinities, commercial candies that contain egg.

Table 7.12
MILK-FREE DIET

Food Group	Foods TO Eat	Foods NOT to Eat
Beverages	Fruit juices, carbonated beverages, water; coffee and tea without milk or cream.	Any made with milk or with chocolate cocoa or mixture containing milk or milk products.
Breads	Ry-Krisp, or any kind of cracker or bread made without added milk; rice cakes, popcorn cakes; corn or flour tortillas or tortilla chips.	All bread rolls, muffins, biscuits, doughnuts, popovers, sweet rolls, pancakes, waffles, pretzels, and crackers made with milk or milk products.
Cereals, Grains	Any cereal to which no milk or milk products have been added. Read labels. Serve cereal without milk or cream; fruit juice can be added.	Cereals with milk added. Pastas with milk or cheese added. Read labels.
Desserts	Plain and fruit-flavored gelatins, angel and sponge cakes, fruit ices or popsicles, soy milk ice cream, other desserts made without added milk.	Cakes, doughnuts, dumplings, pastries, commercial sherbets, mousses, ice creams, custards, cookies, pies, and puddings made with milk or milk products.
Fruits, Vegetables	All fruits and vegetables prepared without added milk.	Any fruit or vegetable prepared or served with a sauce containing milk, cream, or cheese.

Table 7.12
MILK-FREE DIET Continued

Food Group	Foods TO Eat	Foods NOT to Eat
Meats, Poultry, Eggs, Fish, Game, Meat Alternatives	Prepared without added milk; scrambled eggs or omelets without butter or margarine. Read labels. Some luncheon meats and hot dogs contain milk products. Nuts, peanut butter, dried peas, beans, and lentils prepared without milk products.	Dishes prepared with added milk or milk products, cheese, or sour cream.
Milk and Milk Products	Soy milk and milk substitutes.	Fresh, whole, and skim milk; cultured milk, buttermilk, creams; condensed, evaporated, dried milk or milk solids; casein and lactalbumin; butter and margarine; curds and whey; powdered and malted milk; all cheeses.
Miscellaneous	All spices, nuts, olives, pickles, popcorn, salt, spices, flavoring, extracts.	Creamed and scalloped foods; foods dipped in milk batter or fried in butter or margarine; foods prepared *au gratin*; prepared mixes for biscuits, cakes, cookies, doughnuts, muffins, pie crusts, and waffles if they contain milk or milk products.

continued on next page

Table 7.12
MILK-FREE DIET Continued

Food Group	Foods TO Eat	Foods NOT to Eat
Salad Dressings, Sauces, Gravies, Soups	Catsup, mustard; gravies, meat and other sauces made without milk or milk products; soups, bisques, and chowders made with water; dressings made without milk or milk products. Read labels.	White, cream, butter, and hard sauces, and any food using these types of sauces; any sauce or gravy made with milk or milk products; soups containing milk or milk products.
Sugar and Sweets	Brown, granulated, powdered, and maple sugars; honey, molasses, jellies, jams, preserves, marmalades; candies made without milk. Read labels.	Commercial candies that contain milk.

Table 7.13
WHEAT-FREE DIET

Food Group	Foods TO Eat	Foods NOT to Eat
Beverages	Fruit juices, carbonated beverages, water, chocolate, cocoa, coffee, tea.	Coffee substitutes and other beverages made from wheat products; malted drink, beer.
Breads	Ry-Krisp, rice cakes, popcorn cakes, corn tortillas, corn bread, and other products made without wheat flour.	All bread rolls, muffins, biscuits, doughnuts, popovers, sweet rolls, pancakes, waffles, pretzels, crackers, chips, or tortillas made with wheat flour.
Cereals, Grains	Any cereal not made from wheat and to which no wheat or wheat products have been added. Read labels. Corn pops, krisped rice, puffed rice, wheat-free pastas.	Wheat cereals and those containing wheat or wheat products. Read labels. Pastas, macaroni, ravioli, mostaccioli.
Desserts	Bavarian creams, cornstarch puddings, soft or stirred and baked custards, ices, mousses, meringues, tapioca pudding, rice pudding, gelatins, homemade ice creams, sherbets, oatmeal, rice or rye cookies made without wheat products.	Cakes, doughnuts, dumplings, pastries, commercial sherbets, ice creams and ice cream cones, custards, cookies, pies, and puddings made with wheat products.

continued on next page

Table 7.13
WHEAT-FREE DIET *Continued*

Food Group	Foods TO Eat	Foods NOT to Eat
Fruits, Vegetables	All fruits and vegetables prepared without added wheat.	Any vegetable prepared or served with a sauce thickened with wheat flour or those prepared and served with breading.
Meats, Poultry, Eggs, Fish, Game	Prepared without added wheat. Read labels. Some luncheon meats and hot dogs contain wheat products.	Swiss steak, croquettes, fish or meat patties or loaves; luncheon meats and hot dogs which contain wheat.
Milk and Milk Products	All products. Read labels. Some yogurts contain wheat as a thickener.	Any product with wheat used in the recipe.
Miscellaneous	All spices, nuts, olives, pickles, popcorn, salt, and spices.	Malt products. Spice mixes containing wheat flour as a thickener. Hydrolyzed vegetable protein (HVP), vegetable protein, modified starch.
Salad Dressings, Sauces, Gravies, Soups	Bottled sauces containing no wheat products; clear bouillon and consommés; any soups made without wheat products.	Cream soups, bisques, chowders—unless made without wheat flour.
Sugar and Sweets	Brown, granulated, powdered, and maple sugars; honey, molasses, jellies, jams, preserves, marmalades; candies made without wheat. Read labels.	Commercial candies that contain wheat products.

References and Suggested Readings

Arizona Department of Health Services. *Nutrition and Pregnancy Guidelines*. Office of Nutrition Services: Phoenix, AZ, 1990.

Breastfeeding Tips, adapted from *Breastfeeding Helper*. Nutrition Council of Arizona Breastfeeding Advocates, 1991.

Dietitians' Patient Education Manual. A.S.P.E.N.: Gaithersburg, MA, 1991.

Diet Therapy vs. Drug Therapy in CVD Treatment, adapted from highlights of the Report of the Expert Panel on Blood Cholesterol Levels in Children and Adolescents, *Pediatrics* 89(3), 1992.

Health and Nutrition Examination Survey I of 1971 to 1974, adapted from A.R. Frisancho, New Norms of Upper Limb Fat and Muscle Areas for Assessment of Nutritional Status. *Am J Clin Nutr* 34:2540, 1981.

Huggins, K. *The Nursing Mother's Companion*. The Harvard Common Press: Cambridge, MA, 1986.

Lawrence, Ruth. *Breastfeeding: A Guide for the Medical Profession*. Mosby: St. Louis, MO, 1989, p. 178.

Mason, D., and Ingersoll, D. *Breastfeeding and the Working Mother*. St. Martin's Press: New York, 1986.

National Research Council. *Recommended Dietary Allowances*, 10th ed. National Academy Press: Washington, DC, 1990.

Pediatrics Nutrition Handbook. American Academy of Pediatrics: Elk Grove Village, IL, 1993.

Possible Problematic Medications During Lactation, modified from *Transfer of Drugs and Chemicals into Human Milk*. American Academy of Pediatrics, Copyright 1989.

Recommendations for Working Mothers, adapted from *Nutrition and Your Child*. Baylor College of Medicine, Children's Research Center, Spring 1993.

Safe Storage Times For Breastmilk, developed by Pat Bull, *Breastmilk Collection and Storage*, Medela, Inc.: McHenry, IL, 1994.

Satter, Ellyn. *Child of Mine: Feeding with Love and Good Sense.* Bull Publishing: Palo Alto, CA, 1991.

Satter, Ellyn. *How to Get Your Kid to Eat, But Not Too Much.* Bull Publishing: Palo Alto, CA, 1987.

The Breastfeeding Answer Book. La Leche League International: Franklin Park, IL, 1992.

U.S. Department of Agriculture and the U.S. Department of Health and Human Services. *Food Guide Pyramid: A Guide to Daily Food Choices.* National Live Stock and Meat Board, Copyright 1993.

Waterlow Classification Chart. British Medical Journal 3:566–569, 1972.

Index

albumin, 63
allergy, food, 65, 86, 89, 105
  egg-free diet, 116–117
  milk-free diet, 118–120
  wheat-free diet, 121–122
anemia, 57–59, 66
anthropometric measurements, 36, 37, 50

balanced meals and snacks, 4, 5, 94–97, 99, 100
biochemical assessment, 36, 37, 55
body fat, 56
bottles, baby, 4, 88
breast pump, 70, 71
breastfeeding, 2, 68–77
  foods and beverages, 78
  medications, 65, 77

calcium, 4, 9, 13, 22, 60
carbohydrate, 61
cardiovascular disease, 6, 62, 106–108
choking, 87, 89
cholesterol, 6, 62, 108
colic, 104
constipation, 104
cystic fibrosis, 65

diarrhea, 104
diet history, 2–6, 36–38

eating disorders, anorexia nervosa, 109–111
  bulimia nervosa, 109, 111
energy, 29–34
  increasing intake, 31, 84, 85, 90, 91, 114, 115
engorgement, 73

failure to thrive, 35, 53, 54, 65, 66, 84, 85, 90, 91

fat, intake, 98, 106, 114
  malabsorption, 62
feeding, adolescents, 109
  infants, 16, 68
  problems, 92–94
fiber, 23
fluid, 32
fluoride, 2, 13
folate, 8
Food Guide Pyramid, 15
food intake, ages birth to 2 y/o, 16–19
  ages 2–4 y/o, 16, 20, 92–95
  ages 5–18 y/o, 16, 21
foods, baby, 30
  infant, 31
  solid, 2, 3, 65, 86, 89
  table, 4
formula, composition, 81–83
  concentrations, 84, 85
  intake, 4, 34
  methods of preparation, 79, 80
  types, 80

glucose, 61
growth, 3–6, 39, 40, 53
growth charts, 39, 41–49

height, 42–49, 55

iodine, 9
iron, 3, 4, 9, 14, 24; deficiency, 57–59, 66

jaundice, 74

lead, 64
lipid, 62

magnesium, 9
mastitis, 75
milk, cow's, 3, 4

niacin, 8
nipples, flat or inverted, 75, 76
nutrient requirements, 32
nutritional risk, 35, 99
nutritional status assessment (NSA), 1–6, 35–38

obesity, 55, 56, 65, 66, 113

phosphorus, 9
physical examination, 36, 37
plugged duct, 77
potassium, 25, 64
prealbumin, 63
preemie, 11, 12, 14
protein, 7, 29, 30, 32, 34, 63

Recommended Dietary Allowances (RDA), 1, 7–10
referral criteria, 65, 66
regurgitation, 105
riboflavin, 8

selenium, 9
snacks, 97
sodium, 26
sports nutrition, 99, 101, 102

thiamine, 8
tooth development, 68, 88, 90
triceps skinfolds, 50–52

vegetarianism, 65
vitamin A, 4, 7, 11, 27
vitamin B_6, 8
vitamin B_{12}, 8
vitamin C, 3, 4, 8, 11, 27
vitamin D, 7, 12, 28
vitamin E, 7, 12, 28
vitamin K, 7, 13
vitamin/mineral supplementation, 1, 11–14, 102
vomiting, 105

Waterlow Classification Chart, 54
weight, 39, 55
weight gain, 2, 40, 53, 70, 84, 85
weight gain, inadequate/poor, 3, 90, 91, 110
weight loss, postpartum, 69
weight-for-height, percent of standard, 54
Women, Infants, and Children (WIC), 66, 67

zinc, 9